The Immune Spirit

The Immune Spirit

A Story of Love, Loss and Healing

SUSAN RYAN JORDAN

Health Communications, Inc.
Deerfield Beach, Florida

www.hci-online.com

Library of Congress Cataloging-in-Publication Data

Jordan, Susan Ryan
 The immune spirit: a story of love, loss and healing/Susan Ryan Jordan.
  p.   cm.
 ISBN 1-55874-924-1 (tradepaper)
 1. Jordan, Susan Ryan, 1939—Health,   2. Breast—Cancer—Patients—
United States—Biography.   I. Title.

RC280.B8 J667 2001
362.1'96994'0092—dc21
[B]   2001039231

Publisher: Health Communications, Inc.
      3201 S.W. 15th Street
      Deerfield Beach, FL 33442-8190

R-09-01

Cover design by Lisa Camp
Inside book design by Lawna Patterson Oldfield
Cover photo by Bill Keefrey, Ft. Lauderdale, Florida

For Pat

They have had a peculiar sorrow, and a special temperament with which to meet it.

—Elida Evans
A Psychological Study of Cancer, 1926

CONTENTS

ACKNOWLEDGMENTS

I wish to thank my publisher, Health Communications, Inc., for having faith in my story and for the gracious help from all there to me. In particular, to editor Allison Janse, who first read my book proposal and championed it; to Erica Orloff, who respected every word of the manuscript; and, most especially, to my editor, Christine Belleris, who from the day I began to write it, nurtured and protected my story and helped me to shape this book.

My thanks to Kim Weiss, Maria Dinoia and Randee Feldman for their support and enthusiasm in promoting my book.

Thank you, Gaylen Goins, my expert and patient "computer tutor" for showing me how to unravel the mysteries of the computer.

Thank you to all the volunteers of Reach to Recovery of The American Cancer Society for their gifts of hope and inspiration, to me and all of those who have had breast cancer.

"When you are ill, do not be depressed, but pray to the Lord and He will heal you. Then let the doctor take over—and do not let him leave you, for you need him."

ECCLESIASTICUS, 38:12.

I wish to express my gratitude to the gifted plastic surgeons who helped me to mend my body. Dr. Gary Mombello, of New Haven, Connecticut; Dr. Claude J. Noriega of Miami, Florida, and Dr. Vernon Turner of Fort Lauderdale, Florida.

My deepest thanks to the two doctors who cared for me in that frightening time when I had breast cancer. To Dr. Bernie Siegel, who first explained to me that the mind can heal the body and who then encouraged me to care for myself.

And last, but most important, to Dr. William B. McCullough, my surgeon, who became my friend. Bill, although you might not have known, you calmed my terrors, and renewed my hope in those dark days. In all the bright years since you have always been there for me. Thank you.

PROLOGUE

I wake in the middle of the night to the sound of my parents whispering to each other. There is something frightened in their voices. In the dim light of my bedroom, I look across to my little brother's crib. He is sleeping. He's two years old. I am five. Everything in our room seems to be as it should be. My wooden dollhouse with the pink roof is on the table under the window. On the other side of the window is my brother's playpen, and next to that is the big green armchair where my mother sits and reads to us. In the corner of our room is my grandmother's old china cabinet, which my mother has painted yellow and filled with our toys and books. My dolls sit in a row on the middle shelf, staring down at me as always. Suddenly my mother runs into our room. She snatches me out of bed and carries me under her arm over to my brother's crib. She grabs him up under her other arm.

She hurries with us out of our bedroom, down the narrow hallway into the dining room. She shoves us under the dining room table.

"Stay there," she tells me.

"Why?" I ask.

"Shhh!" she says.

She goes quickly through the darkness, past the light of the half-opened bathroom door toward her bedroom. I can see her struggling to help my father move something big through their bedroom doorway. It is the mattress from their bed. They carry the mattress into the dining room and lay it on top of the table.

My brother and I often play under this table. It has fat, round legs, and it's long and made of dark wood. It used to belong to my mother's Aunt Mamie, who lived in England. Sometimes my mother throws a sheet over the table and my brother and I make believe that we are in our own tent, like the GIs I hear my parents talking about at night when I am in bed. I wonder if she'll throw the sheet over the table, but she doesn't. She crawls under the table with my brother and me.

My father has turned off the bathroom light. Now I hear him in the kitchen pulling down the shades over the windows, which look over the back courtyard of our apartment building. The children who live in our apartment building play in the courtyard. We have swings there and a sandbox. Poplar trees and a tall hedge surround the courtyard and a black iron gate leads to the Avenue in Queens, New York, where we live in this spring of 1944.

My father comes out of the kitchen and hurries past us in the darkness into the living room. He pulls down the venetian blinds that cover the three big windows behind the sofa. He crosses to the window over the bookshelves where he keeps his yellow and white *National Geographic* magazines and his books with the pictures of old sailboats. He pulls the blinds down over that window, too, but he opens just one slat and looks through it, out and up into the night sky. I can hear the faint droning sound of approaching airplanes. Under the table, my mother pulls me and my brother up onto her lap. Her arms tighten around me so that I can hardly breathe. Her breath comes in short gasps. My father crawls under the table with us.

"What's the matter?" I ask them. I am starting to be afraid.

This droning sound of the airplanes has lulled me to sleep every night since I can remember. At night, after I am in bed, I hear my mother and father in the kitchen talking about the planes . . . the B-52s, they call them, the bombers that fly over to Europe to help "our boys" win the war against Hitler. My father has taken me to

Idlewild airport near where we live to see the planes. They're big brown planes that lumber down the runway and take off into the sky far above our apartment house. These are the planes that keep us safe. It's the B-52s, our bombers, that make the droning noise. Isn't it?

"What's the matter?" I ask again.

"Shhh!" my father whispers, sharply.

The sound of the planes grows louder and louder. The noise is like thunder over our heads. The floor seems to be shaking. The noise feels like it is inside of us. My little brother screams in the blackness. I break free from my mother and try to crawl away from her, to run over to the window, to look out, to see what my father was looking at up in the night sky. But my mother grabs my foot and drags me back under the table. She wraps her arms around me again. I struggle to free myself from her, to get away from her, to get out from under this table where I can't breathe. But she won't let me go. Finally, the sound of the planes starts to fade. The noise grows dim and far away, and then there is quiet, and darkness and the sound of my mother's short breaths.

The next morning, when my father talks to the woman who lives in the apartment next to ours, he learns that the wailing air raid siren that awakened him and my mother was the all-clear signal and not the alert. He tells my mother that we were the only family in the building who had crouched in fear, in the darkness, waiting for German warplanes that never came.

"I hope they don't tell anyone," my mother says. "What will people think of us?"

I ask my mother why we had hidden under the dining room table.

"It's the safest place to hide," she says.

"To hide from what?"

"If they were German planes, they might have dropped bombs on us."

"But they weren't," I say.

"They might have been. You never know what might happen."

Several nights later, I hear the sound of the planes again. This time I don't wait for my mother to come into the bedroom for my brother and me. I am already up, running for the front door to our apartment. I must get us out of here! I will run down to the basement of the apartment house where there will be a deep, dark place for us to hide. We will be safe there. But the door to our apartment is locked. I can't get out! I shake the doorknob and beat on the door. I scream and scream for someone to help me open it. My father runs down the hall toward me. He picks me up. I struggle violently to get away from him but he carries me back to my bed. "No! No!" I am still screaming. It is only after the droning sound of the planes overhead has faded away that I can stop. But I know that nothing is safe anymore. I can't escape the fear of what might happen. I have no control.

CHAPTER ONE

Cancer

Thirty-five years later, on a November night in 1979, I lay in a darkened room of Yale-New Haven Hospital in New Haven, Connecticut. That night, I heard the eerie, muted sing-song calls for doctors over the intercom. I heard the hushed voices of the night nurses and their soft, quick steps outside in the corridor. But of all the sounds in the hospital that night, the worst was the muffled weeping of the woman in the bed next to mine. The sound was full of terrible and unspoken loss, fear and desolation. I was lying in the bed next to the door. Her bed was next to the window. She had turned her head very far away, almost into her pillow, trying to hide the sound of her grief.

She'd been admitted several hours after I was, and she had not spoken a single word, not to the nurses who came to attend her, not to her doctor who came by to see her, not even to her family who had gathered around her bed earlier that evening to visit her and bring her comfort. Instead, she lay with her eyes closed tightly as if trying to block out everyone and everything around her, as if to shield herself from some inevitable calamity that was about to happen. But she couldn't protect herself. She had breast cancer. So did I.

I looked around. *Another darkened room,* I thought. Another night of terror. But this night, there were different sounds. Not the sounds of airplanes rumbling overhead while I, a child of five, crouched, terrified, under the dining room table. No. On this night, the sounds were of stifled sobbing and anguish in a sterile hospital room. There was no one to protect us. There was no deep, dark place to hide until the danger passed away. The danger was here. The calamity had come.

Early the next morning, my breast would be cut off. There was no escape from this. Like the woman next to me, I was powerless, alone, terrified.

ৡৢৡৢৡৢ

My torment had begun three weeks before, in Bethel, Connecticut, on a brilliant October afternoon when I went to see my gynecologist about a lump I had in my right breast. I'd had the lump for several years and had it checked regularly, but on this visit I saw a look of concern on the doctor's face as he felt it. "What's the matter?" I said.

"This doesn't feel the same," he said.

I felt a sudden sharp stab of fear, then panic. "What do you mean?!"

"It feels hard. It's rooted in there. I'd have a surgeon look at it as soon as you can."

I left his office and drove home. I was a teacher at Choate Rosemary Hall, a boarding school in nearby Wallingford, and I lived on the campus. On my way home, I pulled into a gas station near the school. I wanted to call Pat, a man I'd met several months earlier, who had urged me to see the doctor.

He was the only other person who knew about this lump in my breast. I hadn't told my four children. I'd been divorced from their father for three years. My oldest daughter, Dana, nineteen, was living in California. My daughter Peggy was a freshman at the University of Connecticut in nearby Storrs. She was eighteen. My two youngest children, Andrew, fifteen, and Annie, thirteen, were going to be students at Choate. Andrew was still living with his father. He would come to the school the next year. Annie lived with me in one of the faculty apartments in the freshman girls' dormitory. I didn't want her to overhear my conversation with Pat when I told him about my visit to the gynecologist. I could hear the concern in his voice when I said I had to see a surgeon about the lump.

"What does your doctor think it is?"

"He didn't say," I said. "Do you know of a surgeon?"

"No. Can you ask someone at school?"

As soon as I got home, I called Dianne, one of my new friends who taught with me in the English department. She gave me the name of the dean of breast surgery at Columbia Presbyterian hospital in New York. The man was a pioneer of the Halsted radical mastectomy, an operation in which the entire chest muscle is cut off with the breast, leaving the chest wall caved in and hollow. He didn't believe in the success of the new modified version of the amputation. Pat went with me into New York to see him.

He was a tall, thin, old man with a shock of white hair. I remember thinking how long his arms and legs were. In his white coat, he reminded me of a large stork. When he felt the lump he shook his head. I saw a look of fury pass over his face, and he muttered something I couldn't hear.

Of course I needed a biopsy, he said. He would perform it in the operating room and wait there for the results while I lay anesthetized on the operating table. If the biopsy should be positive, he would perform his operation then and there. He would slice off my breast and my chest muscle without my even waking up. I would have no say at all.

"But I won't have any choice," I said. I felt as if I couldn't breathe.

The doctor raised his eyebrows and stared at me.

"If you have cancer of the breast, of course you have no choice." he said.

He shook his head, astonished at my ignorance. I gasped. I slid off the examining table and stood up.

"I have to get out of here!" I said to him.

He looked at me, curiously. "Suit yourself," he said. Then he turned and stalked out.

I got dressed and rushed out to the waiting room and over to Pat who was standing by a window.

"What?" he asked, alarmed. "What happened?"

"Let's get out of here," I said.

We went to the elevator and pressed the button for the main floor. Inside the elevator I told Pat what the man had said. I began to cry.

"What's the matter with him?" he said, incensed. "Of course you have a choice! It's your breast! You don't have to stay here."

Outside, the sky was overcast and the air was humid, oppressive. We drove through the city streets over to the East Side in silence. A light rain had begun to fall, and the streets were slick, shiny. Pat turned to me.

"If this should be a dangerous thing in your breast, it can be cut out. Once it's gone you'll be well again. I know it. We'll get a second opinion."

I nodded. I looked out the window at the rain and the gray buildings looming over us. I didn't believe him.

꩜꩜꩜꩜꩜

Choate's health plan included the doctors of The Surgical Associates of New Haven, three surgeons who practiced at Yale-New Haven Hospital and taught at Yale. They were Richard Selzer, Bernie Siegel and William McCullough. I made an appointment to see one of them early the next week. I drove down to New Haven after my classes on the following Tuesday.

I sat for several minutes in the waiting room of their office until a nurse appeared and showed me down a hallway past several closed doors and into an examining room. She laid a little white paper jacket on the examining table.

"Take off everything from the waist up and slip this on," she said. "Leave the front open." She patted my arm and left the room.

I took off my blouse and bra and put on the little paper jacket. Then I sat down on the examining table to wait. I felt naked, sitting there. Alone. A strange, ringing noise had begun in my ears, and I felt suddenly lightheaded and nauseous. Again, I felt I couldn't breathe. *Oh, God,* I thought. *What is happening to me?* I tried desperately to calm myself. After all, I told myself, this is Yale. These doctors must be highly skilled. If anything was wrong with me they would certainly be able to cure me. And besides, at least now maybe I had some kind of choice.

The door opened, and the doctor strode in. He was tall, in his early fifties, and he had the lean energy of older Ivy League men who are still athletic, like the coaches at school. He wore loafers, chinos and a light blue, oxford cloth shirt under his white coat. He put his hand out to me. "Dr. McCullough," he said. His voice was deep, calming.

"Susan Ryan."

"Good Irish name," he said and smiled at me. "What's going on?"

I described the lump and how long I'd had it.

"Let's take a look."

As he felt the lump, I searched his face for any look of concern but he gave no sign of what he was thinking. Instead he pulled a chair over from the side of the room and sat down in front of me. His eyes were kind, gentle.

"I can see that you're worried and I understand why," he said carefully, "but this is small. There's a good chance it's nothing serious but I would like to do a biopsy." He smiled at me again, reassuringly. "What do you teach at Choate?"

As we began to talk and I saw how kind he was and how genuinely interested he was in me and what I taught, I relaxed for the first time in weeks. He didn't seem to be that worried about the lump. Maybe the disaster I feared was not about to happen after all. And maybe the fatigue that had depressed me for months would finally go away. It was a certain kind of fatigue, a constant ache in back of my eyes, that made me feel drained, hollowed out, empty, exhausted. Maybe now I would finally be able to sleep. I made an appointment to have the biopsy the next day and left the office.

Pat drove up to New Haven from Fairfield to wait for me in the surgeons' office while Dr. McCullough did the biopsy. It was a quick, painless procedure. Almost too easy, I thought. When it was over I went out and sat down next to Pat in the empty reception room to wait for the result.

We sat thumbing through magazines. Pat kept trying to interest me in an article he'd found about dogs, but I couldn't concentrate. It wasn't that I was thinking of anything else. It was as if I was suspended in that room with its plain linoleum floor and hard yellow plastic chairs forced to wait . . . for what? I tried to make an effort to be interested in what Pat was saying. I took the magazine from him but my hands were trembling and I dropped it. He leaned over to pick it up and gave me a sideways look.

"I'm sorry," I said. "I'm very cold."

"Try not to worry," he said. He put his arm around me.

At that moment, Dr. McCullough burst into the waiting room and rushed over to us. He looked shocked.

"Susan, I think you'd better come in to my office," he said to me. He looked at Pat and then at me.

"It's okay," I said. "This is Pat. This is my friend."

Pat stood up to shake the doctor's hand. He'd come straight from his office, and he hadn't changed his clothes. As a writer, he'd worked in a solitary room for so long that he paid no attention to what he wore. Sometimes he worked in his pajamas. Today he wore ripped jeans, flip-flop sandals and a red T-shirt with an image of Superman on the front of it. The doctor stared at Pat and then at his T-shirt. He seemed not to notice Pat's outstretched hand. He looked back at me.

"I'm afraid it's not good news," he said.

We followed the doctor down to his office and sat down in two chairs facing his desk. I remember that as I sat there it seemed to me that I was watching a play that was about to begin. The characters were all in place for the opening scene. There was the doctor in his white coat, sitting behind his desk, one hand to his forehead. There was the younger man with the dark curly hair, in his red T-shirt, leaning anxiously toward the doctor. Finally, there was the pale, thin woman with long, dark brown hair and frightened, light blue eyes. She wore a brown tweed skirt and a beige silk blouse. She sat, straight and rigid, in her chair in front of the doctor, her hands locked together in her lap. As I watched, the scene began to unfold and I heard the doctor's voice. He spoke slowly, and his words seemed long, drawn out, distorted, as if coming from the far end of a long tunnel.

"The tumor is malignant. You have cancer. The cancer is aggressive," he said.

I heard the dark-haired man's voice.

"Can't it be something else?" he asked. "Can't it be a mistake?"

I saw the woman turn slowly in her chair and look at him.

"No," she said in a flat voice. "It can't be anything else."

But it was my voice.

The surgery was scheduled for the end of the following week. I could not have imagined how long that week would be. On the way out of the office, the nurse gave me a book that one of the other surgeons, Dr. Siegel, was referring to all the group's patients. The book was called Getting Well Again by a cancer specialist, Carl Simonton, his wife Stephanie, a psychotherapist, and James Creighton, a cancer caregiver and counselor.

Outside in the parking lot, I tried to reassure Pat. I was calm enough to drive back to Wallingford by myself. He must drive back to Fairfield, I said. He had to get back. His wife and children wouldn't know where he was. And I had to get home. I had to think of some way to tell my children that something was wrong.

I made sure he drove away before I got into my car. I sat there for a few minutes to control my shaking legs. I looked around the parking lot. It was a brilliant October afternoon, but the sunlight was harsh, glaring. The red and gold of the autumn leaves were too vivid, gaudy, against a sky that was too clear, too blue. The other cars and buildings around the parking lot looked surreal, shimmering in the strange, garish light. I remember feeling oddly calm, sitting there in my car, in spite of my trembling legs. I felt satisfied somehow, as if a private prophecy I'd made about myself had finally been fulfilled. I had always been terrified that I would get breast cancer. I'd lived in fear of it, but I had expected it at the same time. The truth was that I believed I deserved it. Now I had it. Now I no longer needed to fight my fear. I could rest. Now I felt as if the ordeal of the past years of my life, the guilt, the fear, the helplessness of all those days was finally over. I looked at the book in my hand. Getting Well Again. Sure, I thought. Who gets well again from cancer? I started my car and drove home.

CHAPTER TWO

The Loss

We, however, are caught,
Tormented by what is past
And what is to come.

SENECA

Early that evening I told Annie about the small lump in my breast. Just a small lump, I said. Only a few days in the hospital. Routine surgery. I'd be home and fine in no time. I called Andrew and his father and then Dana in California. I left a message with one of Peggy's roommates to have her call me. I never mentioned the word cancer. I couldn't bear to have my children worry about me. Here they were, soon to be in a new home, in a new school, making new friends. They were all starting new lives. How could I do this to them? How could I take all this away from them? How could I take myself away from them . . . again? But I pushed that thought to the back of my mind.

Late that night in my study I tried to concentrate on the day ahead. My classes started early the next morning. I taught in two departments: English and Theatre Arts. I was planning to talk about the Roman playwright, Seneca, in the History of Theatre class that I taught with the head of the drama department. I'd translated some of his writings in Latin class in high school. As I sat reading through my notes I came across a passage from one of his essays.

> *Wild animals run from dangers they actually see*
> *And once they have escaped them*
> *Worry no more.*
> *We, however, are caught,*
> *Tormented by what is past*
> *And what is to come.*

What is to come? I wondered. *I have cancer. I can't escape this. I'm caught. Trapped.* For the first time, I allowed myself to think about what the doctor had told me that day and a nauseating fear swept over me. What if the cancer was spreading? What if it was moving through my body, taking it over, even as I sat there at my desk? How could I stop it? What if it was invading my liver? My lungs! How would I breathe? My brain! How would I think? How would I know? What if an operation was useless? I remembered my mother's words: "You never know what might happen." But this had happened! If only I, like the animal, could escape! But where could I go?

Cancer. It was a word that I'd heard said only in whispers all my life. I could remember my mother and her sisters talking about some-one who had just died of the disease. I could still see them, usually so lighthearted, sitting at the kitchen table, sighing, shaking their heads sadly, closing their eyes. "She never had a chance," they would whisper. "It spread before anyone even knew he was sick." "There is no cure." Cancer. The word meant certain death.

God! I thought, *Help me!* I tried again to calm myself, to control my fright. I grabbed for the book Dr. Siegel's nurse had given me. I saw that it was about the authors' work with cured cancer patients. Cured cancer patients? You weren't cured of cancer. The only way you got rid of cancer was to have a doctor cut it all out. Then, if you were lucky, you lived a while longer. But, finally, it killed you.

I began to read anyway. "If you have cancer," the authors wrote, "take a piece of paper and list any major life changes or stresses that were going on in the six to eighteen months immediately prior to the onset of your illness." They urged the reader to pay particular attention to the loss of a close relative, a divorce or a separation from one's family or the loss of an important goal in life. The cancer patients, they said, had described feelings of hopelessness and helplessness in the face of this loss. In the cancer patient, this despairing emotional response triggers a set of physiological responses that suppress the immune system and make it unable to fight off illness, in particular, the growth of abnormal cells. The authors seemed to suggest that cancer is somehow associated with the way certain people react to loss. I put the book down. I had endured all of the losses they described, all at the same time, just eighteen months before.

In the late autumn of 1977, two years before, I had divorced my husband of seventeen years. We had married young. I was nineteen; he was twenty-one. Over the years, our marriage had become empty and silent. My loneliness and his indifference to me caused a quiet strain that I could not understand or resolve. He wasn't surprised or unhappy at my decision to divorce him, but he told me that if he had to rent an apartment for himself he couldn't continue to pay the mortgage on the house for the children and me. We had bought it with a down payment given to us by his father. If he had to move out, we'd have to sell the big, comfortable house, and the children would be uprooted and miserable. He wouldn't be able to give me child support, not on his math teacher's salary. If he left the house, the children would suffer the loss of their lifestyle. If I left, they wouldn't.

He begged me to let him stay in the house with the children . . . just for a little while, just until I "got on my feet," as he put it. Since I was the one who wanted the divorce, I should be the one to leave, he reasoned. He didn't want it. The children didn't want it. If I left the children would suffer less. *I* should be the one to leave. I believed my husband. I agreed to leave.

In those days, it was expected that a woman put her husband and her children's needs before her own. In my generation, a woman lived to please others. If your marriage was troubled you never burdened anyone else with your problem. I never asked anyone else for advice or for help for myself. I had no money of my own, no livelihood, no sense of control. I believed my husband when he said he couldn't give me alimony. I believed him when he said any money he gave me would come out of my children's mouths.

Why didn't I believe that I was more important to my children than the house they lived in? Why didn't I insist that my husband move out? Why didn't I take them with me? Then, I didn't know the answers to any of those questions. In my confusion and guilt, I left them. I caused all the anguish yet to come.

I went with nothing but my clothes and an old, green Ford Pinto. I drove to the next town and stayed with friends for several months. It was November, too late to apply for a teaching job at any of the area high schools. I had already applied for a position at Choate Rosemary Hall, a nearby boarding school, but the person I was to replace didn't retire. I had no money. I believed my husband when he said he couldn't afford to give me any. The only work I could find was as a substitute teacher in several of the local high schools for twenty-five dollars a day. But even teaching three days a week, I couldn't earn enough to meet my basic expenses.

Nightmares tormented me. The dream was always the same. There was an empty, wooden house with tall, vacant windows. I stood in front of it as a yellow school bus rolled up and stopped. My four little children came out of the house, and I helped each one of them climb into the bus. I watched as they took their seats and waved to me, smiling. Then the bus started to move away from the house, down the driveway. But suddenly my four children appeared in the back windows of the bus. Their anguished faces were framed in the back windows. Their eyes were terrified. They were sobbing, reaching out to me, begging me, soundlessly, to take them off the bus. It was a silent image, like an old photograph, frozen in time. In the dream, I ran wildly after them but the bus picked up speed. As fast as I was running, it stayed just ahead of me. I couldn't catch it. Then it moved faster and faster, until it was only a small yellow dot far down the road . . . too far away from me. And then it disappeared.

I woke from the dream drenched in sweat, struggling for breath, not knowing that I had been screaming in my sleep. The room was strange to me until I saw the anxious faces of my friends in the doorway. I tried to block out the last frame of my dream, tried to keep myself from sobbing. If I allowed myself to cry, I might never be able to stop.

I could not sleep at night, and in the days I worried desperately about money. I didn't know whether I could support myself. I became more and more anxious. One of my friends was an actor. Seeing my desperation, he suggested I try out for a part in a TV commercial that would pay me residuals. Then I could at least pay my bills. He introduced me to his agent, and I made one commercial for Hills Brothers coffee that ran for the next year and eased some of my financial distress. The casting director for the commercial needed an assistant. I grabbed the job. I moved to New York temporarily, and lived in a succession of sublet apartments borrowed from actor friends who were out of town on tours. I worked long days for the casting director, and I moved constantly from one strange apartment to the next.

I talked to my children almost every day by phone and took the train up to Connecticut to see them every weekend. But I believed that I could never see them enough. Back in New York and alone in those borrowed apartments, I fell into exhausted sleep. And every night I had the dream. I woke and pushed my tears back, constantly, so much that my throat ached. Were my children as heartbroken as I? I believed they could never forgive me.

Then my mother died. She had been crushed by my decision. To her, a devout Catholic, divorce was a mortal sin and a social stigma. She couldn't understand why I had left my children. She was heartsick for them and mortified by me. I had been excommunicated from the church. I was an outcast. I had disgraced her and betrayed my children. She began to complain of a pain in her back, and then she was dead, within three months, of lung cancer. It was unbelievable to me that she could die, that I would never see her again or hear her voice. I was convinced that I had killed her. No one could have told me that I hadn't.

During those long months alone in New York, every time I thought of my lost children and my dead mother I felt a physical pain, a pang in the upper part of my stomach, then panic. I was the selfish one who wanted the divorce. I'd betrayed every trust, as a mother and daughter. I had hurt everyone I loved and disappointed them profoundly. My guilt was overpowering. Crushing.

I came to believe that I had nothing left to live for . . . that I shouldn't be living. I began to believe that I had no control over what was happening to me, that I was helpless to change the course I had set for myself. I became filled with a deep sense of hopelessness and dread. My greatest fear was of breast cancer. I thought that would be the way I would die. But it would be a relief to die, I thought. That would be the way out. The escape. The fitting punishment. The loss of my breast would be the price I would pay for my sins of omission as a mother and a daughter. The loss of my life would be the sacrifice for the people I had failed.

Now I had it. Breast Cancer. Here I was, two years later, sitting, panic-stricken, late at night in my study at Choate. My self-fulfilling prophecy had come true, and in spite of the fatigue, the curious emptiness I felt whenever I thought about the future. Now I desperately wanted to live, to make a new life for myself and my children. Was it too late? If only I, like the animal, could worry no more! If only I was not tormented by the past, I thought. And what was to come?

CHAPTER THREE

The Immune System and the Mind

That night in my study, I read on and on, trying to find some answer in the Simontons' book. It had been published the year before, in 1978. Dr. Siegel had met the Simontons in June of that year at a teaching seminar in Portland, Connecticut, where they gave a workshop called "Psychological Factors, Stress and Cancer." He would later write that his entire practice of medicine changed as a result of meeting the Simontons and that workshop. I know that what I read in their book that night changed my life.

Psychologist Stephanie Matthews Simonton was interested in "unusual achievers"—exceptional people who are highly motivated to achieve success. At the same time, her (then) husband, Carl Simonton, M.D., a radiation oncologist, became fascinated by certain of his "terminal" cancer patients who were still showing up for their yearly physical exams years after they were expected to have died. These were people who had literally defied every medical expectation. When Carl questioned these former cancer patients and asked them to explain their good health, they all said that they refused to die because they believed they had many goals they wanted to accomplish. They believed that they could reverse the course of their disease, and they did: they'd healed themselves by taking control of their thoughts and changing their outlook. Every one of these healed former patients found a new psychological strength and a powerful, positive self-image. They were no longer victims of their own fears and anxieties.

I realized that I was reading about a revolutionary kind of healing whereby patients were working, with their physicians, to heal themselves. They were "participating" in their cures. They were unusual achievers who had somehow regained the will to live. How had they done this? I read on, fascinated. The authors explained that a living being must be considered as a harmonious whole. This was a view shared by ancient physicians, who believed that the mind and body are intricately connected. The Simontons explained that our bodies actually change when we react to a certain event. I thought about this for a moment. Why do our palms sweat when we are apprehensive? Why do we blush when we are embarrassed? Why did my hands tremble in the waiting room of Dr. McCullough's office while I waited for the results of the biopsy? Apparently my anxious thoughts produced those certain changes in my body.

According to the authors, the immune system is also affected by anxious thoughts and emotions. When the immune system is functioning in a healthy, normal way, its powerful, vigilant cells seek out abnormal invaders in the body, in particular, weak and confused cancer cells. These powerful immune system cells find the cancer cells and kill them, leaving other organs in the body to flush the dead, diseased cells out. This "search out and destroy" process takes place continuously and automatically when the immune system is functioning properly, going about its business, destroying the abnormal cells that are occasionally present in everyone.

But when the normal process of the healthy immune system is disturbed by stressful, anxious thoughts or feelings of grief and despair, the brain releases certain chemicals that suppress the immune system and keep it from functioning in a normal way. This breakdown allows the cancerous cells to grow.

The Simontons' research with recovered cancer patients showed that positive feelings of hope and expectancy cause the brain to respond instantly, creating an array of powerful hormones and peptides that rush to the immune system and buoy it, making it strong and vigilant, enabling it to overcome the illness. The authors insisted that if the patient could change feelings of helplessness and despair to feelings of hope, control and optimism, the course of cancer could actually be reversed. Amazingly, when the Simontons' patients took control of their thoughts and began to believe that they could recover—expected to recover— they began to overcome their feelings of despair. They became hopeful and peaceful; they found the will to live again and their cancers disappeared.

I wondered. Could we really control our immune systems by taking control of our thoughts and changing them? And once the immune system is strong and vigilant, could it destroy the cancerous cells? And did Dr. Siegel, a respected surgeon used to cutting cancer out of people, also believe, as the authors did, that the mind and the body and the emotions are not separate from each other, but work together to heal the whole living being?

But how? And could we be in charge of our own healing? The Simontons seemed to suggest that if the patient could gain a new perspective on his or her problems, make a decision to change the way events are viewed, overcome the emotional despair and find a hopeful outlook, the course of cancer could be stopped.

I sat back. The book seemed to be about changing one's view of events. I thought back to my recent emotional shocks. The events were traumatic, certainly. And they'd all been related to loss. But the events of the last eighteen months had not been hopeless in themselves. My great stress had come from the way I'd perceived the events. Why had I viewed the shocks and losses as hopelessly as I had? A quotation I'd once read from the Talmud came to me: "We do not see things as they are. We see them as we are."

I knew that each of us learns certain attitudes and beliefs in childhood that determine how we "see" or perceive an event—with more or less anxiety, helplessness and fear than others. Now I understood that I had been a captive of my own anxious perceptions all my life. To survive, I had to overcome my guilt and change the way I viewed the things that happened to me. I had to find some faith in the future. "God," I said out loud, again. "I have to change the way I think! How?"

"Many things which cannot be overcome when they are together yield themselves up when taken little by little," wrote Plutarch. That was it. I remembered that the first step toward overcoming fear is finding a sense of control. I'll control these anxious thoughts one by one. I'll think of the most hopeful thing instead. I'll think about tomorrow! I made myself concentrate on the lesson plan for my first class in the morning. I finished that and then the plans for all my classes the next day. Then I went to bed. Annie and I had to be up on time. Both of us had an early class.

∾ 𝒢 ∾ 𝒢 ∾ 𝒢

Choate Rosemary Hall is a great, old New England prep school, one of the most venerable and prestigious boarding schools in America. Its graduates go on to Yale, Harvard, Princeton, Dartmouth.

Some go on to Oxford and Cambridge. They become world leaders and influential financiers, authors, entrepreneurs. The school numbers, among its more illustrious graduates, John F. Kennedy, Adlai Stevenson, Edward Albee and John Dos Passos. The campus, set in the rolling hills of rural, northeastern Connecticut, looks more like an idyllic New England village than a school. Ancient oak trees hang over the white clapboard colonial houses and ivy-covered brick school buildings. At the very center of the campus, surrounded by sweeping green lawns stands the chapel, modeled after a typical New England church, its graceful, tall, white spire rising up against a background of gentle, wooded hills.

I'd first seen the campus several years earlier, months before I was divorced, on a gray February morning when the place was knee-deep in snow. I'd never forgotten the ethereal peace and security of the place. I'd always dreamed of teaching there, and I'd wanted my children to be students there. But by the time I finally became a teacher there, my two older daughters, Dana and Peggy, had already graduated from high school. My son, Andrew would attend the following year. Annie and I lived in a spacious apartment on the ground floor of the freshman girls' dormitory. Two hundred freshman girls lived in the building with three other faculty families who, like me, were "house parents." The building was isolated, built on the far side of one of the wooded hills that surround the main campus. I loved the peaceful, pastoral setting.

In the days right before I went into the hospital, I was thankful for the busy school-day routine. Life at the school barely allowed any free time, but that was fine. I didn't want to have time on my hands to think. My classes began at 8:00 A.M. and my last class was over at two in the afternoon. I taught in two departments, English and theatre arts, so I carried a heavier class load than some of the other teachers, but I didn't coach an after-school sport as most of them did. After school, I met with students who asked for help on the essays that I assigned once a week.

I was thankful for the rigors of Annie's classes, too. Every minute of her day was filled with schoolwork, then homework. After school, she was required to play some sport, either crew, soccer, track or swimming. She was overwhelmed at first. Some nights she fell asleep hours before lights out at ten o'clock. But every so often, I caught her looking anxiously at me. At thirteen, she was tall and awkward, all long arms and legs. Her long, dark brown hair was a mass of curls. She had her father's clear, green eyes.

One afternoon after school she said to me, "Mom, you aren't going to die, are you?"

"Not now, for goodness sake," I said.

I was torn. Should I tell her the truth about the lump on my breast? No. She had been through enough anxiety. I was determined to make her life as normal and full as I could. I had vowed to try to make her calm. I was glad that we lived in the freshman girls' dormitory and that she was surrounded by her friends and the other faculty families. The only people at school who knew why I was going into the hospital were the dean of faculty and my friend, Monica, a fellow English teacher. Her husband, John, was a resident doctor at Yale-New Haven Hospital. Their apartment was down the hall from ours at the dorm, and Monica would watch out for Annie while I was in the hospital.

For me, the nights were the worst of that awful week before I went into the hospital. I tried to make myself as busy those nights as I was during the day. I had rounds at night to make sure all the girls were in bed by ten. Then, after Annie was in bed and asleep, I immersed myself in lesson plans for the following day and then, exhausted, went to bed. But I always woke before dawn as if from a deep sleep, looked at the small alarm clock next to my bed and saw that I'd slept for only two or three hours. I tried to remember why I felt vaguely anxious, uneasy, in the middle of the night. Then I would realize that

I carried cancer in my breast. The fierce reality shocked and terrified me just as if I was hearing the diagnosis for the first time. The fright swept through me and overwhelmed me just as I was waking . . . when I was least prepared to face it. I saw myself lying dead in a white, satin-lined coffin surrounded by baskets of flowers and tall candles. The image horrified me. I didn't want my casket to be open before my funeral mass. I didn't want my children to see me dead! Where would I be buried? I didn't know. Who would take care of all these things? Should I? When?

I jumped up quickly, as if to flee the bed, the terrible thoughts and those dreadful questions. I stumbled out to the kitchen and made coffee at two or three in the morning to keep myself awake, so that I would not want to go back to that bed. I found the small, normal routine of brewing the coffee comforting. Then I hurried into my study, grabbed my books and notebooks and buried myself again in the lesson plans for the day ahead.

I began to dread going to sleep at all. To calm myself at night, I read more of the Simontons' book before I went to bed. One night, just before the end of that week, I came to the pages describing mental imagery and how people can use their imaginations to visualize their own recoveries. This was the most fascinating reading of all.

The Simontons had decided to study the psychological techniques that Stephanie used in her work with her highly motivated "unusual achievers." They wondered if by using these techniques of mental imagery, positive thinking and biofeedback, gravely ill cancer patients could achieve positive attitudes of hope and control.

Biofeedback especially interested them. This technique enables people to influence their own internal body processes, such as blood pressure and heart rate, by visualizing these processes and then using mental imagery to control them. The Simontons hoped that by using this same "visual imagery" process their patients could participate in their own recoveries.

They outlined a program during which the patient, in a period of relaxation, visualizes the cancer in some imagined form, then the treatment that is destroying the cancer. Next, the patient visualizes the body's natural defense system as it surrounds the cancer cells, destroys them and carries them off. The patient visualizes the body finishing the job by flushing all the dead and dying cells out through the liver and kidneys. They instructed their patients to perform these visualizations three times a day. After four years of study of the "incurable" cancer patients, the Simontons discovered that those who used their imaginations to visualize their own recoveries survived twice as long as the patients who received medical treatment alone. They realized that the more vivid the mental imagery was, the more effective was the visualization technique.

One night I decided to construct my own mental visualization. First, I made myself concentrate on relaxing all the muscles in my body, starting at the top of my head and going all the way down to the soles of my feet. Next, I imagined sitting alone at the beach on a quiet afternoon, with no noise but the sound of the smallest waves. Then, I imagined the small, black cancer cells, those I was most afraid of, that were huddled in my breast. Then, as I had read, I visualized the powerful white cells of my immune system mobilizing, all through my body, forming armies to look for the cancer cells. Then I imagined the armies of powerful white cells finding the cancer cells, wherever they were, sweeping over them and destroying them all. I thought of my immune system cells as fighters and defenders, watching over my entire body and caring for it. Last, I imagined the strong and victorious white cells sweeping the dead cancer cells up and carrying them to my liver and kidneys so that my body could flush them out. At the end of the exercise, I added my own final steps. I got up and drank a tall glass of water . . . just to hurry the dead cancer cells out quicker. Then I made up my own experiment. I took a deep breath, as if to fill myself with hope, and while I held it, I thought of the most wonderful and hopeful thing that had happened to me during that day. I promised myself that during those minutes of hopeful breaths I would not think of anything other than the day I would be well again. From that night on, whenever I thought about the cancer in my breast I imagined my immune system finding the cancerous cells and killing them. I held on to that thought for as long as I could. Sometimes I lay in bed and swore out loud at the stupid cells.

Toward the end of the week, I noticed that a strange thing was happening. Whenever I felt a fearful, anxious thought about my breast cancer, I pushed that thought out of my mind and made myself concentrate only on my schoolwork. I thought ahead to the goals I had to accomplish. They were small goals, but goals nonetheless. I simply had to reach the end of each class, then each lesson plan, each day. I was in charge. I was controlling my thoughts. I reasoned that every positive thought I had was helping my immune system fight to help me. At night, the mental imagery exercises I did were the second step in getting well again. Maybe I could use my own power to fight the disease!

Pat came up to Choate to have dinner with Annie and me the night before I went into the hospital. He knew I wanted to stay calm for Annie's sake, and she loved his company. We walked down the hill from my apartment to the main campus dinner in the dining hall. This was an ivy-covered, brick building near the chapel at the center of the campus. Just outside the door was the usual crowd of strollers and tricycles belonging to the children of faculty families, knapsacks belonging to students, tennis racquets and lacrosse sticks leaning against the wall. Inside was a long room with high ceilings, dark wood paneling, tall-paned windows and polished wood floors. A huge fireplace with an ornate, wood-paneled mantelpiece took up the entire far wall of the room.

The hall was noisy with sounds of many voices and laughter, the din of clattering plates and silverware, and the scraping sounds of chairs being pulled up to the dining tables. Faculty families and students ate together in captains' chairs around the large, round wooden tables. Although there wasn't a uniform for the teachers at the school, they all wore the same thing. The men wore blue oxford shirts with the sleeves rolled up, loosely knotted ties, rumpled khaki pants, blazers and topsider shoes. The women wore blazers, too, but with long pleated skirts, prim, white blouses and loafers. This day, Pat wore a World's Gym T-shirt with a picture of a gorilla lifting a heavy barbell. He had on sneakers and a pair of faded jeans. He was a big man, broad-shouldered and muscular, with dark, curly hair, and the dark stubble of a beard. After dinner, one of my colleagues from the arts department came up to us as we were leaving. "Not only do you look like you don't belong here," he said to Pat, "But you look like someone no one here should even know." Then he burst out laughing.

"Ask me if I care," said Pat, and he let out one of his rare, big, hearty laughs.

Then he took out a cigar from the shoulder bag he always carried and lit it. He hadn't noticed the faculty staring at him. His only concern was that Annie and I felt calm on this night. He put an arm around both of us as we walked with him to his car.

"Did your mother give you my office number?" he asked Annie.

She nodded, yes.

"Remember, I told you I'll take you to see her whenever you want," he said. "And don't worry." He kissed us both good-bye and got into his car. "I'll try to call you later," he said to me. "Promise you won't worry."

Annie and I walked together through the early evening darkness, across the campus on our way back up the hill to our apartment. It was early November and the chill night air was damp. We crossed over the wooden footbridge that spanned the pond next to the Arts Center. A mist had formed over the pond. It hovered in wraith-like shapes over the surface like a crowd of thin, gray ghosts. We passed through the empty courtyard of the Arts Center toward the flight of stone stairs at the far end that led to the path up the hill. From the bottom of the stairway the hill wasn't visible. All you could see was the stairway that led up to a vast, empty sky. I remember feeling a strange sense of foreboding as we climbed the steps. I saw Annie glance at me anxiously as I stared up at that sky. She put her arm through mine. "Mom, what are you thinking?"

"Nothing," I said. "Nothing at all."

CHAPTER FOUR

Yale-New Haven Hospital: Day One

I walked into Yale-New Haven Hospital before dawn the next morning, on November 9, 1979. I didn't want to tell the nurse who admitted me why I was there. I was afraid of the look on her face when I said the word. But, of course, I had to tell her. She looked up from my paperwork and stared at me without expression.

"Of what?" she asked.

"Excuse me?" I said.

"Of what?"

I couldn't answer her.

"Cancer of the what?" she said. "I have to put it down."

"Oh," I said. "My breast."

"Which one?"

"My right breast."

"Oh," she said, and she wrote that down. "How old are you?"

"Forty."

"Give me your left wrist," she said.

"Why?"

She didn't answer. I put out my left wrist. She snapped a plastic bracelet on it. My name and some other letters and numbers were typed on it.

"What's this for?" I asked.

Annoyed, she looked up at me again from her paperwork. She stared at me for a long moment.

"In case you can't speak," she said.

Upstairs, the room I was given had four beds. Two were next to a double window, which provided a clear and expansive view of the sky. This was the first bright note so far. My bed was next to the door, but I could see the blue sky, and on this day, some high, wispy clouds drifting by. My nurse was a big, blonde matronly woman who introduced herself as Rita. Her white, starched nurse's cap looked like a tiny white sailboat riding on upswept waves of her bleached blonde hair. She gave me a plastic bag for my clothes, including my underwear. She laid a thin cotton patient gown on the bed. The gown had a faded but cheery nursery print of little flowers and rabbits, which looked ridiculous. She told me to leave the back of the gown open. Someone would be taking me downstairs shortly for a CAT scan, she told me. "Not to worry," she said. "It's just an x-ray of your whole body."

The technician in charge of operating the CAT scan was as kindly as my nurse had been upstairs. "Sometimes people get a little scared," he said, "but I'll talk to you on your way through, if you like. Just remember to lie perfectly still." As I went through the dark tunnel of the CAT scan, I remembered to try to control my thoughts. The machine was like a long, silver tube, huge, awesome. I felt closed in, trapped, powerless inside it. It could look inside of my body and see parts of it that I would never see! What if it found cancer everywhere? I felt the fear rising again and a throbbing, thumping sound in my head. But then I remembered what I'd read in the Simontons' book: Every change in the mental state is accompanied by a change in the body. A bad thought affects the body. "So, don't get your mind upset," I said, out loud, to myself. "You don't want your body to look crazy."

"Okay in there?" asked the technician from outside.

"Okay," I said. But what would the machine find?

Back in my room, the day went on toward afternoon. An anesthesiologist was supposed to come and talk to me about my operation, scheduled for early the next morning, but I still hadn't seen him or Dr. McCullough. I tried to keep myself occupied with some reading that I'd brought from school. I called Annie and Andrew several times and talked to them about anything that was usual. How had Annie's classes gone that day? What was Andrew doing on the weekend? I called Peggy at her school, but I still couldn't reach her. I was leaving a message for her when Dr. McCullough came into the room.

"I've ordered another CAT scan," he said. "There seems to be a slight abnormality with your liver."

I couldn't even think what the "abnormality" might be. What did all this mean? Why hadn't I seen the anesthesiologist? What time was my surgery tomorrow?

"I'd like to wait to see what the new scan shows. If there is a problem in your liver we might want to think about an alternative treatment rather than the surgery," he said.

An orderly came and wheeled me back down to x-ray where the hulking CAT scan machine sat by itself in the middle of the dim room. Alone in the dark tube for the second time that day, I began to feel curiously angry. *I hate this!* I thought to myself. *I'm not worrying anymore. I've wasted enough time worrying.* I grew furious. "Get out!" I said to the invisible cancer in my breast. "Get the hell out."

In my room, I watched the sky outside the window turn to deep violet and then to black. It still had not occurred to me that the cancer in my breast might have spread to my liver. I was too tired to think. I closed my eyes and slept.

The stifled sobbing of the woman in the bed next to mine woke me again, much later. I tried to think of something I could say to her to calm her, to let her know she wasn't alone. I was afraid. She was afraid. How much easier it would be if we could comfort each other . . . whisper to each other in the darkness about our fears. Maybe they wouldn't seem so overwhelming. But I hesitated to intrude on the solitude she had wrapped around herself. What could I say? What could I say to anyone with this disease? What could I do for her? For myself? Was I facing death in spite of all my efforts? If only I could escape this thing that would happen in the morning!

I looked around the dark room. I saw myself again as the little girl I was on that long ago night, crouched, terrified, under a dining room table, waiting for bombs to shatter everything around me while everyone else in our apartment house slept peacefully in their beds. I have felt helpless for as long as I can remember, I thought.

I remembered the quotation from the Talmud again: "We do not see things as they are; we see them as we are." And then I understood that the journey I'd made to this hospital bed had begun when I was a little girl. My anxious, fearful perceptions had been formed in those days of my childhood. I realized that the helpless lessons I'd learned so long ago had been more crippling than the loss of my breast could ever be. To live, I would have to go far back to remember those teachings, and once I remembered and understood them, I would have to put them aside.

Where would I begin? I remembered Plutarch's words again, "Many things that cannot be overcome when they are together, yield themselves up when taken little by little." That was the answer. I would go back to my earliest memories and try to overcome each fearful, anxious lesson, one by one.

~~~~~~

My mother gave birth to me on a hot August morning in New York City in 1939. Her labor had been long and painful. She had suffered for twelve hours when her doctor went out to my father, who was waiting anxiously down the hall. "The baby is in a breach position," he told my father. "Your wife is extremely weak. I don't want to do a cesarean section because the baby is too far along. I am afraid I won't be able to save them both."

My mother told me that moments before I was born she lost consciousness. She saw herself as if from above, lying on the delivery table, and then she heard her dead father's voice calling to her from across a wide river that she could just barely see. "Peggy!" he called. "There is nothing to be afraid of. It's very beautiful here. Come on!" Then she heard the voice of the doctor saying, "No, Peggy. You have a beautiful baby girl. Come on!" Then she heard me crying. She told her father, "I have to go back, Dad." Then she woke up. My mother told me that I became her reason for living. She told me that story for years. She never changed a word of it.

A month later, in September 1939, World War II broke out in Europe. By the following year, Hitler dominated most of Europe, except England, which the Germans bombed mercilessly, day and night, for months on end. Americans watched nervously as the war in Europe raged. Then, on December 7, 1941, the Japanese attacked the U.S. Pacific fleet at Pearl Harbor in Hawaii, killing thousands of Americans. The next day America declared war on Japan and entered into the World War that we would fight for the next four years.

My earliest memories were of the sounds at night in those years and the feelings of uncertainty and fear. From my bed, I could hear the war news on the kitchen radio and the names "Roosevelt" and "Hitler"; the sounds of the big B-52 bombers that rumbled over our apartment house on their way to Europe, and always, every night, the sound of the long, rising wail of an air raid siren . . . the sound of fear and warning. I remember that at night the venetian blinds were always drawn over our windows.

We lived in an eight-story "garden" apartment building called Griswold Hall in Jackson Heights, then a leafy suburb on Long Island. The building was red brick and had an elaborate, curved white marble arch over the double front doors. In back, the building had two wings, one on each side, with a garden courtyard in between. We lived on the second floor, in the middle of the building, overlooking the courtyard. My father paid fifty dollars a month in rent, expensive in those days, but by then he had started working for The Revere Copper and Brass Company in Manhattan, where he was in charge of pricing the metals used for the guns and bullets we used in the war. This job was part of "the war effort" and kept him, for the first few years at least, out of the war.

My mother's older sister, Emily, had stopped dancing as a Rockette at the new Radio City Music Hall in Manhattan and married a handsome young man who worked as a radio announcer for NBC. They lived next door to us with their young son, my cousin. My mother's older brother, Tom, had joined the Navy and was serving in the South Pacific. My mother's youngest sister, and my godmother, Lucille, had just left her job making bullet casings for the war effort and joined the American Red Cross. She was to be stationed in North Africa. I remember the day before she left to go overseas. It was late April 1942 and my two aunts came with my grandmother to see my mother, just home from the hospital with my new baby brother. My aunts wore short, flowered dresses, high-heeled shoes with open toes and had flowers in their upswept hair. They laughed together around the kitchen table, each one taking a turn holding my baby brother. My new brother was a wonder to me. I sat next to my aunts and gazed at him. I touched the softness of his fine, dark hair and one of his tiny hands. His baby fingers curled around one of mine. That afternoon, when my mother put him back to sleep, I sat next to his crib for hours and watched him as he slept. I would watch over him for all the years of our childhood.

At night, after supper, in those days, my parents listened to the radio in the kitchen as they did the dishes together. They listened to "Fibber McGee and Molly" and "The Bickersons," with Don Ameche and Frances Langford playing a constantly bickering husband and wife. They listened to Frank Sinatra, the new young singer from Hoboken, New Jersey, as he sang, "I'll Be Seeing You" and to Tommy Dorsey play "I'm Getting Sentimental Over You." They sang "You gotta ac-cent-tchu-ate the positive, e-lima-nate the negative and latch on-to the affirmative. Don't mess with Mr. In Between!" When Glenn Miller played "In the Mood," my father would fling the dishtowel over his shoulder, grab my mother around the waist and dance around the kitchen with her until she was laughing and breathless. But then the war news would come on, and they would sit down at the kitchen table, the dishes and their dancing forgotten. I saw fear pass over their faces as the reports of the war came over the radio.

Prime Minister Winston Churchill spoke to the British people: "If we fail, then the whole world, including all that we have known and cared for, will sink into the abyss of a new dark age." My parents were terrified. They sat close to one another at the kitchen table. The entire world was at war. What might happen to us?

My friends' fathers, Mr. Ruppel, Mr. Lyons, Mr. Zavitkovsky and Mr. Messina, were soldiers fighting overseas and so in those war years, the women in our building raised their families by themselves. They gathered downstairs in the lobby at their mailboxes every morning, and while they waited for letters from their husbands who were overseas, they talked quietly among themselves, exchanging news they had already received.

In the early years of the war, my father's job kept him from being drafted, but in 1943 the local draft board called him up several times. My father's heart beat so frantically during the physical exams that he was deferred because of arrhythmia, a suspected heart defect. He tried once to enlist in the Navy, but his racing heartbeat caused him to fail that exam as well. When my father came home from work every night the women would ask him for help with any household jobs they couldn't do by themselves. In my family, our days went by as usual with the set routines that were safe and secure.

I played with the other children in the courtyard in the springs and the summers. We sang in the courtyard as we played "soldier" and "GI": "Over there, over there, the Yanks are coming, the Yanks are coming, and they won't come back till it's over, over there!" We called up to our mothers in the summer afternoons when the Good Humor Ice Cream man came to the courtyard gate. He wore a white uniform and a white cap shaped like a policeman's, and he pedaled a bicycle with a white refrigerated box strapped onto the front handlebars. A raspberry Popsicle cost seven cents. Upstairs our mothers would put a nickel and two pennies into white handkerchiefs, then lean out of the upstairs windows and drop the handkerchiefs down to us in the courtyard below. We children would wait as the handkerchiefs came down like white parachutes and then scramble for the handkerchief we knew was ours.

Before supper I sat in front of the mirrored dressing table in my mother's bedroom while she brushed my hair. Sometimes she'd braid it and wind the braids around the top of my head. Other days she swept it up and fastened it on top of my head with her small enameled combs. If she brushed too vigorously, my eyes would smart. "Never mind," she always said. "Beauty must suffer." She sang to me then, while she stood behind me, brushing my hair, one of the wartime songs, "You'll never know just how much I love you . . . you'll never know just how much I care . . ." Sometimes the war seemed very far away.

Some afternoons my Grandmother Ryan came and baby-sat for my little brother so my mother could take me on the Fifth Avenue bus into Manhattan. My grandmother made a pale blue, light woolen coat for me. It had a deep blue velvet collar and velvet buttons, and she'd found a bowler for me of the same deep blue velvet. She put the coat on me, buttoned it up and adjusted the collar. Then she grasped the coat at the bottom and gave it a sharp tug down with such force that I almost sank to my knees. "There," she said. "Now that's a snug fit. You look quite smart."

My mother wore a tailored, tweed suit and a brown velvet hat with a short veil. We always wore our white gloves. We took the double-decker bus across the bridge over the East River into Manhattan. People sitting near us on the bus would say to my mother, "What a happy, beautiful little girl you have!"

"Thank you," my mother would say. "She is my angel."

In the summer we wore flowered dresses and rode on the open top deck of the bus. We sat on the new woven straw-covered seats of the bus and looked up at the two high arches of the Queensboro Bridge. Underneath the bridge, in the dark, swirling waters of the East River, was Welfare Island and the gray hospital of the chronically ill, but I never noticed those buildings until I was much older. I didn't know that my grandfather, my father's father, was lying in a bed in that hospital even as my mother and I were crossing the bridge high above him. I didn't know that just before I was born he had been transferred there from the Manhattan State Hospital for the Insane. I never knew he was alive. I didn't know of him at all until many years later, long after he had died, in that hospital, without ever regaining his mind.

My mother and I got off the bus at Fifty-ninth Street, and walked down Fifth Avenue past the sparkling windows of the Stueben Glass Company and Tiffany's Jewelers and Bonwit Teller department store to Saint Patrick's Cathedral where my father had served Mass as a little boy. We always stopped before going in and looked far up at the tall, twin gothic spires of the cathedral. They looked odd, old and beautiful, like two fairy-tale castles made of gray lace, among the skyscrapers.

My mother was devoted to the Blessed Virgin Mother. It was one of her many beliefs that you could not pass "Saint Pat's" without going inside to the Lady Chapel for a visit. We went into the great, dim, gray church that smelled of melted candle wax and incense and walked up the wide main aisle to the high altar at the front of the church. We genuflected in front of the altar and then went around to the back of the altar into the Lady Chapel. My mother lit two votive candles in front of the white marble statue of the Blessed Virgin. "This way she'll always take care of us," my mother said.

"Why?" I would ask.

"There's a war on. You never know what might happen."

Then we'd go out onto the busy avenue again and walk down to Saks Fifth Avenue where my mother bought our white gloves: a pair for her and a pair for me. Further down the avenue, we went into Best and Company where Mr. Paul cut my hair. After lunch at Stouffer's Restaurant, we walked across the avenue to Rockefeller Center. We walked through Rockefeller Plaza, past the six shallow pools with their bronze fountains to the skating rink with the huge golden bronze statue of Prometheus. We'd go around the rink and over to Radio City Music Hall where my Aunt Emily and my Aunt Grace had danced as Rockettes. If we had time we'd see the afternoon matinee: a movie and, of course, the stage show. My aunts' friend Mr. Crangle still played the huge Wurlitzer organ there. Sometimes we met my father after his work and the three of us rode home to Jackson Heights together on the bus. Later, after supper, I could hear my parents talking about the day and the city, but always their talk turned to the war.

My mother used war ration stamps when she shopped for groceries at the Safeway or at the butcher shop. Without them she couldn't buy any rationed goods. Beef was rationed. So was pork and bacon. She needed the stamps for butter, cheese, canned fish and even milk. The stamps came in long, thin booklets and were imprinted with pictures of tanks, airplanes, submarines and machine gun caissons.

On the front of the ration booklet, the government had printed an important message. "When you have used your ration, salvage the tin cans and waste fats. They are needed to make munitions for our fighting men. Cooperate with your local salvage committee." Every night before dinner my mother would open one end of the tin cans, empty the contents into a bowl, then open the other end of the can. Then she put the can on the floor and stamped on it to flatten it. At the end of each week my father took all the flattened cans down the street to the local salvage depot.

In the spring of 1944, the war in Europe and the Pacific raged even more furiously. My mother and father were anxious, jittery. The war news was on the radio every night. The announcers talked of "D-day" and "Eisenhower" and "Omaha Beach." After I was in bed, I heard my parents' hushed voices in the kitchen, talking of German U-boats and submarines sailing close to New York and of German bombers "blitzing" Manhattan. Every night our bombers rumbled overhead, and the air raid siren cried out its warning. The women who gathered around the mailbox every morning didn't laugh with each other now. Their men were young husbands and fathers, far away in distant countries fighting, giving up their lives, to keep us safe. Their wives waited silently now for the mailman then took their letters and went quickly back to their apartments. In our apartment, my mother was silent and my father was nervous and preoccupied. Sometimes very late at night, I would wake and hear my father moving around our apartment, from window to window, pulling down all the venetian blinds.

On Christmas 1944, when I was five, almost all of the men in our apartment were gone, fighting overseas. My father put up the make-believe fireplace of cardboard with red bricks painted on it. My brother and I believed that Santa Claus came down through this into our living room, and we pinned our stockings to it. That year my father found a little Christmas tree that my mother put up on the dining room table. That was the Christmas that I heard my parents talk about "the Battle of the Bulge" and "Hitler" and "Berlin" and "the Allies." Mr. Zavitkovsy had been shot in his leg while fighting in France, and he came home. He was very sick. My mother and the other women in the apartment took turns bringing supper to Mrs. Zavitkovsy, and my father stopped at the Safeway market most nights to shop for them on his way home.

After that Christmas, my father began to be more and more impatient with me when I talked about my friends' fathers who were in France fighting, and how I hoped they could stop the Germans and Hitler. "Why can't she be quiet? Why is she such a chatterbox?"

"She's just saying what she thinks!" said my mother.

"Why can't she keep what she thinks to herself? Maybe other people don't want to hear it."

My father became angry at my mother if she spent too much time with us when he was home. "You see them all day," he said to my mother. "Can't you talk to me, instead of them?" I would hear them argue behind their closed bedroom door. "Why are you so hard on them?" my mother asked. "They'll think you don't like them."

"Why do you always think of them first?"

"They're children!"

I began to get up early in the morning when I heard my father get out of bed. I dragged a chair into the bathroom and sat down and watched as he filled the sink with water to shave. I watched as he swirled his shaving brush around in the wooden box of shaving creme to make a lather that smelled of lavender. He brushed the lather on his face and dipped his silver razor into the sink. He shaved first one side of his face and then the other in long, smooth strokes from his ear down to his chin. He jutted his chin out toward the mirror and shaved his neck. When he finished, he stood in front of the mirror and turned one side of his face to the mirror and examined it carefully, then the other. He ran the tips of his fingers slowly over both sides of his cheeks. Then his eyes met his reflection in the mirror, and he stared at himself for a long moment. He studied his finely chiseled face and looked into his own beautiful, dark blue eyes as if to see what lay behind them. One day he said to me, "Why are you watching me?"

"I love you, Daddy. I like it when you're happy," I said. "I don't like to make you mad at me."

I started first grade at Saint Joan of Arc School, run by an order of French nuns. The school uniform for girls was a gray jumper, a white long-sleeved blouse and a gray beret. In those days, the boys still wore gray knickers and long socks. They wore starched white, long-sleeved shirts, black ties and gray, schoolboy caps. I walked to school every morning with my cousin Mary who was just my age. Her mother was my mother's older sister. They walked behind us pushing their baby carriages down the tree-lined street as we skipped along in front of them. Mary and I wore our berets to one side as our Aunt Lucille had taught us. "All the girls in Paris wear them that way," she said. "With panache!"

In the schoolyard before classes began each morning, the school bell rang and the school monitors, eighth-grade girls and boys, gathered us little ones into straight lines according to class. Boys stood on the left side of the line and girls on the right. The monitors clapped their hands once for silence. Over the loudspeaker came the rousing music of John Philip Sousa's "Stars and Stripes Forever." The monitors clapped their hands twice, and we marched into the school building. At the front double door of the school, the line divided and the boys filed in to the left, the girls to the right. Mary went to a different classroom. Saint Joan of Arc School did not allow members of the same family to be in the same class together.

There were twenty-five girls in my class. We sat in five rows, five girls to a row, facing the front of the room and a raised platform on which sat Sister Imelda's desk. A tall wooden cross with the figure of Jesus nailed to it hung on the wall in back of her desk. Class began every morning with the recitation of the first three questions and answers from the Baltimore catechism: "Who made us? God made us;" "Why did God make us? God made us to know him, to love him and to serve him in this world so that we can be happy with him in the next;" "How do we serve God? We serve God by following his Commandments."

Our wooden desks had tops that you lifted to store your books, notebooks and pencils. The top of each desk had a small, empty inkwell in the upper-right corner, but as first-graders we were not allowed to use pens. Only when you were promoted to the third grade were you allowed to use a pen. In first grade, we learned to write according to the Palmer method, shaping the letters of the alphabet into long, graceful curves. Sister stood in front of the class and passed out pieces of ruled, white paper to the girls who sat in the front desks. We passed the paper over our left shoulders until each of us had a clean, white sheet on our desk. We waited until Sister clapped her hands together once, then we began to copy the letter she had written on the front blackboard. Sister walked up and down each aisle, between the rows of our desks to look at our work. On the first day, she stopped at my desk and laid her hand on my shoulder. I looked up at her. "Now, dear. Don't be frightened." She took the pencil gently out of my left hand and laid it down in the little groove at the top of the desktop.

"Susan, the left hand is the devil's hand. We must learn to write with our right hand, dear. Pick up your pencil and begin again."

"Yes, Sister." I picked up the yellow pencil and tried to hold it between my right thumb and my forefinger. I forced the tip of the pencil onto the top blue line of the paper and snapped the lead. I looked up at her again.

"That's all right, dear. Did you bring another pencil?"

"Yes, Sister."

"Good. Take it out and begin again."

I lifted the desktop to get my pencil case and tried to take out my other new pencil, but my hands shook so that I couldn't unzip the case.

"That's all right, dear. Take your time."

As soon as the school bell rang at the end of the day, we gathered our coats and sweaters and berets from the cloakroom at the back of the classroom and formed a neat line to wait for the dismissal bell. Then we filed outside to the schoolyard where eighth-grade boys were clapping erasers. Puffs of chalk dust covered their hands and faces and settled into their hair, and we could hear them laughing as they blew the chalk dust at each other. My mother waited for me at the entrance to the schoolyard with my little brother and my new baby sister in her carriage. Then we walked home again under the tall trees that lined our avenue.

I adored gentle Sister Imelda. At home every day after school, I sat at the kitchen table and forced my right hand to make the same graceful L-shapes and S-shapes that she drew on the blackboard. My name was especially hard to write because of the letters *a* and *n*, but I spent hours filling sheets of paper trying to write my name without my pencil wobbling. After several weeks at school, I brought home a penmanship paper with a gold star pasted on it and the words, "Lovely work." I don't know why, but my mother saved that paper for years.

All the girls who attended St. Joan's marched in the May crowning procession. That year I was chosen to be the flower girl who would lead the procession. I would march in front of the eighth-grade girl who placed the crown of flowers on the head of the statue of the Blessed Virgin Mother. The scent of lily-of-the-valley and lilac mingled with the smell of incense in the huge church as the girls, all in white dresses, took their places. Organ music swelled to signal the start of the procession, and I could see my mother smiling at me from her seat on the aisle where I would pass. I walked slowly down the center aisle of the church as I had practiced . . . right step, then together, left step then together. I held a big basket filled with rose petals and, as we walked, I took them from the basket and scattered them down in front of the girl who carried the flowered crown. My mother scooped some of the petals up after the procession had passed her pew. She saved those, too, for years. Why? I've often wondered. Maybe in my small successes she saw ones she wished she had achieved?

In the early spring of that year, 1945, our men were fighting furiously in the Pacific against the Japanese. I had made a friend, Chloe, in the first grade. One day she didn't come to school. She was out for a week. Sister Imelda announced one morning that Chloe's father had been killed on the island of Guam. I told my mother at dinner that night. My father interrupted.

"Do we have to talk about this now?" he said.

"I feel sorry for Chloe and her mother," I said. "Sister Imelda said that her father was very brave. He was fighting for our freedom, and he gave up his life."

"I told you to pipe down!" my father said. His face grew red and his voice became shrill. I was afraid he would lose his temper. Then he would spank me.

"Can't she talk about anything else?" he said to my mother.

"But it's all she hears!" she said.

"Shut her up! I hear about this all day. I don't want to hear it at night!"

In the spring of that year, 1945, my father was called up to the draft board again, but this time he was told to report to Grand Central Palace on Lexington Avenue in the city. Reports on the of an all-out push by the Allies to end the war, and every able man was to be drafted into the army. My father left early on a weekday morning to report.

Grand Central Palace was a huge building in the heart of Manhattan, originally intended for exhibitions. On this day, there was an enormous collection of power boats. The scene inside the building was chaotic. As the men arrived, they were told to remove all of their clothing except their underpants and their hats. They were each given two hangars for their clothes, but there was nowhere to hang the clothes. Crowds of men, wearing only their Fedora hats and their underpants, milled around uncertainly, holding their shoes and their clothing. No one knew where to report. They were packed together and pushed up against the power boats. Finally my father was given a physical exam. His heart beat so wildly that he was deferred. He got dressed, went out of the building and into the street, found the first public telephone and called my mother. At home, my mother answered the telephone. Her face was ashen.

"Oh my God!" she said and began to sob.

"What happened?" I said. But she only sobbed louder.

"Why are you crying, Mommy?"

"Your father doesn't have to go to the war," she said.

"Then why are you crying?"

"Because he'll be embarrassed that he was frightened. And then he'll be angry." I was too young to realize how well she knew my father. She knew he couldn't control his fear.

The war ended in Europe in May 1945. Three months later, the United States dropped the atomic bomb on Hiroshima. We celebrated "V-E Day" and "V-J Day." The children cut off the tops of cereal boxes and sent them in with twenty-five cents to receive "an atomic bomb ring." The ring was plastic and had a small round plastic knob with a tiny peephole on the top. You looked into the peephole and saw a mushroom-shaped cloud.

Just after the war ended, two children, a girl, Natasha, who was my age, and her little brother, Peter, came to live with Mr. and Mrs. Fialkoff, the older Jewish couple who lived on the fourth floor. The children's hair was a strange color, dusty looking, almost white. They were shy and very thin, and they held tightly to Mrs. Fialkoff's skirt. They did not speak at all. My mother told me that when the war ended Mr. Fialkoff went over to Europe to search for his relatives. He found Natasha and Peter by themselves in a "displaced persons" camp. Their parents had been killed. The two children were the only members of the Fialkoff family that were left alive. The idea that their parents were dead, their home vanished and they were alone in the world horrified me.

My birthday fell in August. That year my mother decorated our apartment with red, white and blue bunting and American flags. She invited Natasha and little Peter to my party. They came into our apartment clutching each other's hands. They sat quietly in their chairs at the dining room table and watched as the other children laughed and played with the party favors, ate candy from colorful little paper baskets and waved tiny American flags at each other. They stared silently at my birthday cake and shook their heads shyly when my mother offered them a piece of the cake with ice cream. After the cake and ice cream, we began to play pin the tail on the donkey. As my mother put a blindfold on one of the children, I saw Natasha's brother put his hands up to his face in horror. He began to cry, soundlessly. I saw Natasha slip her arm around him and pull him even closer to her. I went out to the kitchen to get my mother. She stopped the game and led the terrified little boy into the kitchen with his sister. Then she took them quietly back upstairs to Mrs. Fialkoff.

Who knows what the sight of that blindfold caused Peter to remember? Who could imagine the sights that little boy and his sister had witnessed? My family had been terrified of bombs that never fell. But the war had destroyed everything for Natasha and Peter. Their terrors had been real.

The men in our building came home from the war, and our families all gathered in the courtyard in the early evenings in spring or went to Jones Beach together on summer weekends. Most Sunday afternoons we had dinner with my grandmother at her house on Ithaca Street in nearby Elmhurst. She always turned the kitchen radio way up so that out in the backyard she could hear the Dodgers baseball game. She sat at the big round table and poured iced tea with wedges of lemon and sprigs of fresh mint from a big, frosted glass pitcher. My father sat in a lawn chair under the tree in the corner of the yard and read the Sunday newspaper. My brother and I sat and sipped our tea with Grandmother as she listened to Red Barber call the game. "Tut, tut," she said after any bad play by her beloved team. "By jingo, they'll lose."

"Why?" we asked.

"It's mind over matter. They're not using the brains God gave them."

While my grandmother sat in the yard, my mother and my aunts went in and made Sunday dinner. They turned the phonograph in the living room way up so that even in the kitchen they could hear the Gershwin songs they loved. Emily and Grace would link their arms and dance together down the length of the kitchen flinging their long legs out, first to the left, then to the right in high-precision kicks. My mother would lean back against the counter and watch them, smiling. She loved those Sundays. My father usually stayed out in the yard. He liked "peace and quiet."

At home, my mother and father had started to talk in the evenings about moving to California. Mr. and Mrs. Zavitkovsky and their children had already moved to Santa Monica where Mr. Zavitkovsky found a good job with a company that was making airplanes. He told my father that California was a place of "wide, open spaces" where the children could grow up, out of the city, with a beautiful beach and the Pacific Ocean nearby. He told my father that he would help him find a job with his company.

In the second grade I was to make my first confession and receive first Holy Communion. We girls and boys practiced for months to receive these two sacred Sacraments of the church. Our teacher, Sister Marie Therese, went over and over the questions and answers in the Baltimore catechism.

"Who made us?"

"God made us."

"Why did God make us?"

"To know him, love him and serve him in this world so that we can be happy with him in the next."

"What is a sin?"

"When you know something is wrong and you do it anyway."

"What is a mortal sin?"

"A terrible offense against God."

"What is the punishment for a mortal sin?"

"We lose our immortal soul and suffer in the fires of hell for all eternity."

We learned the absolute importance of making a good confession. If you confess your sins to the priest and tell God you are sorry for them you will be saved from Hell. Never lie to the priest. Never be afraid to confess the worst thing you have ever thought or done. It is a mortal sin to deliberately omit a sin from your confession. Always tell the priest every sin, even if you aren't sure it is a sin. We sang:

Before you humbled, Lord, I lie
My heart like ashes, crushed and dry,
Assist me when I die.
Full of tears and full of dread
Is that day that wakes the dead,

Calling all with solemn blast
To be judged for all their past.

We learned the responses for the Mass of Absolution and Burial: "Deliver me, O Lord, from everlasting death on that day of terror when the heavens and the earth will be shaken. As you come to judge the world by fire I am in fear and trembling at the judgment and the wrath that is to come."

My Grandmother Ryan made my white first communion dress. I practiced saying the Act of Contrition and the Latin prayer the priest would say before he placed the sacred wafer on my tongue. On the Friday night before I was to make my first confession, I was drying the dishes after dinner. I heard my father and mother, sitting at the kitchen table behind me, talking about the trip to California, as they did almost every night now. I was very nervous about making my first confession. What if I couldn't think of every sin? Would it be a sin if I forgot to tell the priest something? I turned around quickly and blurted out, "Mom, what if . . ."

"Interrupt me again like that and I'll give you a good wallop!" snapped my father.

"Why are you always so mad at me, Daddy?" I said. I started to cry.

My father got up from his chair. He came toward me. Without thinking, I took the butter knife I was drying and held it up. I waved it at him.

"Leave me alone!" I cried.

He sat down and stared at me.

"Well," he said. "Now you really have a good sin to tell the priest tomorrow. Don't forget to tell him what you just did to your father."

That night I was afraid to fall asleep. What if I died before I got to confession? I would go straight to hell. But what, exactly, was I supposed to say to the priest? The next afternoon, I waited with all my classmates on the side aisle of the church to go into the dark little box and tell the priest my sins. My turn finally came. I pushed aside the heavy, red velvet curtain of the confessional and felt around in the dark for the kneeler. For a moment, I was horrified that I wouldn't be able to find it. I would have to go back out into the church without having made my confession! What would people think? As my eyes became used to the darkness, I saw the kneeler and the carved wooden screen that the priest sat behind. I knelt down and the little screen slid open. I could see the side of the priest's face. I felt my heart pounding. I began as I had been taught.

"Bless me, Father, for I have sinned. This is my first confession."

"Yes, dear," said the priest.

"I waved a knife at my father."

"Oh?" said the priest. "Really? What kind of knife?"

"A butter knife, Father."

"Why?"

"I thought he would hit me because I interrupted him and my mother when they were talking."

There was a pause.

"Do you think interrupting is a bad thing?"

"Sometimes, yes," I said. "It means you're not thinking of other people first. I didn't mean to be bad! My father said I had to tell you about the knife!" Now I started to cry. "Is interrupting a sin, too, Father?"

There was a very long silence. I was afraid I would not be able to breathe.

"No, it is not," said the priest, finally. "How old are you, dear?"

"I'm seven, Father."

"God knows you're a good girl. He wouldn't want you to worry anymore." There was another pause. "For your penance, say five Hail Marys. And say a good Act of Contrition."

I went out of the confessional and sat down, dazed, in the pew with the rest of my classmates. Sister Marie Therese came up behind me and tapped me on the shoulder.

"Susan, you're supposed to kneel when you say your penance."

"Yes, Sister," I said. I knelt down and put my forehead on the pew in front of me, exhausted.

A year later, in the spring of 1947, my father bought a new, navy blue Ford sedan. I was eight, my brother was five and my little sister was two. Our apartment was becoming too small for our growing family, and my parents wanted to move further away from the city. They decided to follow many of our neighbors in the Griswold who were moving to Southern California to find better jobs in the booming post-war economy on the West Coast. My father planned to leave his job, put our furniture in storage and drive out to Santa Monica, where we would stay with Mr. and Mrs. Zavitkovsky until he found work. Then we would find a place of our own to live and send for our furniture. We were to leave in the early summer when the school term ended.

On the day my father left his job, my brother and I were laughing, chasing each other, back and forth down the short hall between the dining room and the bedroom. My mother never minded the noise of children playing. But she had taught us to "be still" when my father came home. She always explained that he needed "peace and quiet," especially now that we were planning to move and he was nervous.

This day he came home early. He walked into the hall and grabbed my brother and me by the arm and shoved us ahead of him into our bedroom with such force that we both stumbled and fell down on the floor. "Can't you think of anybody else? Don't you care that I had a rough day?" Then he screamed at me. "You damned brat! You think of yourself first! How selfish can you be?" He took his belt off from around his waist.

He lifted me by one arm into the air and hit me with the belt on the backside, so hard that the flesh on the tops of my legs stung. He hit me again and again so that I swung in the air. He dropped me and kicked me away from him into the table on which sat my dollhouse. The dollhouse and everything inside of it crashed down on me and scattered all over the floor. Then my father turned on my brother. He grabbed him and sat down in the big, green chair that was in our bedroom. He threw my brother over his knees and began to spank him with the belt, methodically, one powerful slap, then another and another and another.

"No!" I screamed. "Stop! Stop it!"

I crawled over to my father and tried to pull on his leg. My mother ran in from the hallway.

"Stop!" she screamed at my father. "They are children! You don't know what it is like to be a child! Can't you let them be themselves?"

My father stood up, and my brother fell to the floor. He stepped over him and stalked out of the room toward my mother. She shrank away from him, but he brushed by her and went into their bedroom. He slammed the door behind him. My mother sat down on the floor and wrapped her arms around us. Out in the kitchen, my sister, left alone in her highchair, was screaming. My brother put his hands over his face.

"Oh, oh, oh," he whispered. He began to rock back and forth, crying softly.

I did not cry. I did not make any sound. This was not the first time my father had beaten us. But it was the worst time.

"It's all right," my mother murmured to my brother. "He doesn't mean it."

"Then why does he always do it?" my brother whispered between his sobs.

My brother and I would not leave the bedroom. It seemed to be the only safe place. We sat close together in the green chair. My brother looked up at me. His face was tear-streaked and twisted with his effort to stifle his sobs. His pale blue eyes were anguished. His body trembled uncontrollably. I put my arms around him. Finally he fell asleep in my lap. Hours later, long past the time we should have been in bed, I still sat in the darkness holding him. I saw my father come to the door of our bedroom. Then I saw my mother appear, right behind him.

"Please leave them alone," she said. "Don't go in there and tell them you're sorry. You're always sorry afterwards. Do you think by saying you're sorry you can take away the hurt?" It was the only time that I remember that she tried to help us, to protect us from our father, but it was too late.

My mother, timid and fearful, always felt safest when someone else was in charge. My father took care of her. She never argued with him, never crossed him, not even for us. She was terrified of losing her security. She understood my father. She knew his fear was a result of his shattered boyhood when he'd lost his home at seventeen. They were both terrified of uncertainty.

CHAPTER FIVE

Fear Is Worse Than Death

Looking back, I understood their terrors. I had inherited them. And here I was, as terrified of the unknown as they had been, laying, helpless, waiting, for what? The woman in the bed next to me had finally fallen asleep. It was very late at night, quiet now, still. There had been no word on the CAT scan, no anesthesiologist, no Dr. McCullough. Nothing. What would the morning bring? How could I know? I remembered a Latin quotation I'd once translated in high school: "The ocean is very deep and wild, but the fear of the unknown is worse than death."

The one thing my parents had in common was their fear. It had controlled them, paralyzed them. Fear was their legacy; learned from their parents before them. Where had the lessons begun? I went further back to remember the stories about my grandfathers . . .

My father's father was an Irish immigrant who came to Manhattan as a young man. There he began a small business as a wood grainer, reproducing the color and grain of real wood on mantelpieces and front doors of the large houses of the wealthy in the city, and he prospered. A photograph taken of him then on Fifth Avenue shows him in front of one of those doors. He's a short, wiry little man wearing a black bowler, cocked over one eye. He looks at the camera with the wary look of a little street fighter. He has a square jaw, a black, brush mustache, high, slashing cheekbones and deep set, dark, brooding eyes.

He met a petite, lively, young German woman, the only daughter of a German family, also newly arrived in America. They married in 1895. My father was born in December 1911 on the top floor of a brownstone house at the corner of Fiftieth Street and Second Avenue, on the east side of New York City. He was the youngest child and his parents' delight. They pampered him in his early years.

In 1921, when my father was ten, my grandfather began to buy property: new apartment buildings on the shore of the East River where the United Nations buildings stand today, which he rented out. When the Great Depression hit in 1929, he didn't evict the tenants who couldn't pay their rent. He couldn't bear to do it, he told my father. The sight of those poor families, sitting in the street, surrounded by their furniture and bags full of clothes was too horrible, he said. And so the tenants continued to live, rent free, in the apartments that he owned. How could he collect money from people who had none? How could he possibly be the terrible landlord who turned them out? What would they think?

Without his tenants' rent he couldn't pay his mortgages. And so one by one, the banks foreclosed on his properties until he had none left. He was so completely shocked at the loss of his money and so afraid of what might become of his family because of his own failure that he suffered a nervous breakdown. At first, he was confined to a private mental sanitarium, but the family's savings, once strong, began to dwindle. His family removed him from the private sanitarium and admitted him to a state institution, the Manhattan State Hospital for the Insane on Ward's Island, a small island in the East River that separates Manhattan from Long Island. When my father was seventeen and in his last year of high school, the money ran out altogether. The bank foreclosed on his family house, and he and his mother were forced into the street.

My father left high school and moved with his mother to Elmhurst, Queens, on Long Island, where he found a cheap apartment and a job to support his mother and himself. He took his mother, faithfully, every weekend for the next ten years to visit her husband, his father, in the mental hospital. They waited in the visitors' room, sometimes hearing the muffled shrieks and cries of the other patients, until my grandfather shuffled into the visitors' room between two nurses. He stared, unknowing, at these two people who had come to see him. My father would look into his father's vacant, dark blue eyes and try to explain who these two people were who had come there to see him. But my grandfather had lost his mind.

In 1939, shortly before I was born, my grandfather contracted tuberculosis in the insane asylum. He was transferred to a hospital for the chronically ill on neighboring Welfare Island, underneath the Queensboro Bridge. I never knew that he was alive when I was a little girl. I never knew that my father went every weekend to visit his father. In all those years, for all those visits, my grandfather never recognized him. He died in that hospital sometime during World War II. My father never told me of his death. But from that time on, my father believed that his father lost his mind because he lost his home. Home, for my father, became his ultimate sanctuary; the only place where he believed he was safe from his fears.

My mother learned her terror of uncertainty from her father. He was the mild and gentle son of English and Irish immigrants who died unexpectedly when he was a young boy. His two older sisters took him in to their house on the East Side of Manhattan and raised him. He entered a seminary after high school to become a Catholic priest, but left before taking any final vows. In 1896, he joined the New York City Police Department. He'd risen to the rank of sergeant when he met my grandmother, Emily Ryan, one fine spring Sunday morning in 1907 when he went to mass at Saint Agnes church, just around the corner from his sisters' house on Park Avenue.

He was impressed by the spirited playing of several of his favorite hymns, and he wanted to congratulate the organist. After mass, he climbed the steps to the choir loft and found a big, handsome woman arranging sheets of music there. Where could he find the talented player, he wondered. "In front of you," she said. They married a year later, in 1908, in Manhattan. Shortly after the wedding they moved to Elmhurst, Queens, on Long Island.

In 1914, my grandfather was promoted to the rank of inspector. I remembered seeing an old photo of him taken then. He wore the distinctive high-collared dark blue tunic of the New York police officer with its double row of brass buttons. His face was fleshy, soft, pale. His eyes didn't meet the camera, but appeared to be gazing past it toward some point in the far distance. His face was expressionless, inscrutable.

He served as a New York City police inspector for twenty-two years and scrupulously avoided any appearance of misconduct. At the height of his career, he was indicted for graft. During his highly publicized courtroom trial, his accuser, a known criminal, suddenly pointed at another policeman in the crowded courtroom as the guilty party, and my grandfather was exonerated. The experience so horrified him that he suffered a nervous collapse. He retired from the police force and spent his last years at home in the house on Ithaca Street. At first he devoted much of his time to his two youngest daughters, my mother and her sister, Lucille, who adored him. But soon he spent more and more time by himself in his room on the top floor.

On the last summer holiday he would take with them, he went for a long walk with his young daughters, along the New Jersey shore. Lucille saw how despondent he looked as they walked.

"What's the matter, Dad?" she asked.

"I can't believe it all happened. I guess you never know what might happen to you. You just never know."

"You must try to forget it, Dad," said my aunt. "You were acquitted."

"Yes, but what difference does that make? There was nothing more important than my reputation. The only thing I had to leave you was my good name."

"What do you mean, leave us?" asked my mother.

"Well," said my grandfather, "I might die soon."

"No, Dad! No!" screamed his daughters.

"Don't worry," he said. "It's just a good, long sleep. At least it's one thing I can count on."

He died several months later, in November 1936. The cause of Grandfather Ryan's death was never fully explained. One member of the family said he had a stroke in his room. Another said he collapsed on the bathroom floor. Still another said he fell down the stairs. My mother said he died of a broken heart. My grandmother never told me how he died.

My mother's suffering at the loss of her father was profound and lasting. She grieved for him, always. I believe he was the great love of her life. She herself died on the same date in November as he had, forty-one years later. She'd watched her father as he slipped from helplessness into hopelessness and then into death. She remembered him as powerless, and she inherited his beliefs. I have always remembered her saying, "You never know what might happen."

My mother never believed in her own power. She was a sweet, quiet girl, who even in childhood photographs looked timid and anxious. In the earliest picture she was eight months old, seated on her mother's lap. She had a fragile, heart-shaped face, wide, frightened pale eyes and straight dark hair. She wore a long, white dress, and she was about to cry. Two older sisters, in lace dresses, stood close behind her on either side of their mother. Her brother, dressed in a white sailor suit, stood next to my mother, one hand resting protectively on her baby foot. Her father was not in the picture.

But he'd always doted on his younger daughter. Perhaps there was something in her fragile nature that appealed to some protective part of him. When my mother was four years old she developed empyema, a dangerous infection, in her right lung and spent one month in the hospital, critically ill. On his first visit to her, he got as far as the doorway to her room. When he saw his little daughter sitting in the hospital bed, still struggling to breathe, surrounded by nurses, he cried out. "Oh no!" he said. "She's too little to be so sick! I can't stand to see her like this!" He fled the sight of her and the hospital.

My mother waited for him every day for the next month to come and see her and hold her, but he never did. She thought it her fault that he had abandoned her, and she blamed herself for his distress. She thought she had failed him because of the illness in her lung. She never believed otherwise. "I made him sad because I was sick," she told me once.

When she got home from the hospital, pale and weak, my grandmother whisked her upstairs to give her a bath and a shampoo. "You smell like the hospital," she told her little girl. "Let's get rid of that memory."

As she began to shampoo my mother's hair, she saw lice crawling on her head. She plucked her out of the tub, dried her off, dressed her and ran out of the house with her, down the street and into the barbershop. "This is Peggy, my daughter," she said to the barber. "Cut off all her hair."

"Why?" said the astonished man.

"She got lice in the hospital. Cut it all off. Now."

The barber cut several inches off the child's hair and then stepped back, as if finished.

"Shorter," said her mother. "Shave it. It'll grow back."

When the time came for my mother to go back to school several months later, she refused to leave the house. Even though her straight, dark hair had grown back nicely, she wouldn't go.

"Why not?" demanded my grandmother.

"What will all the other children think about my hair?" wailed the child.

"They'll think it's short," said my grandmother. "Besides, what do you care what people think? It's *your* hair. Think of it this way! You'll be setting a new style!"

Finally my mother consented to go, but not without an elaborate hat that her aunt knit for her. She was at school for only a few days when she developed a stutter whenever she was called on to read aloud to the class. As the weeks passed, the stutter grew worse. My grandfather suggested that she be tutored at home.

"Nonsense!" snapped my grandmother. "You are spoiling her silly. She must learn to overcome this. It's simply mind over matter." So she practiced reading with her daughter and insisted that she read to the family at dinner every night. "You will not let this overcome you, Peggy. Remember, it's mind over matter!" Finally the stutter disappeared.

Another picture of my mother, taken when she made her confirmation, shows her at twelve, in a white dress, white shoes and stockings. She wore an oversized, enormous bow in her hair, and she wasn't smiling but looking anxiously into the camera. I used to ask her why she looked so frightened. "Oh," she would say. "That picture was taken right before we went to church. I didn't want to go. I was afraid I wouldn't get the responses right and the bishop wouldn't understand me. I was worried that people might laugh at me. But my father told me the bishop would understand if I was nervous."

When she was eighteen and ready to graduate from high school, she volunteered, with several of her classmates, to help clean the auditorium where the graduating ceremony was to be held. While she was sweeping the stage, several of the boys in her class rolled a set of six stairs into the auditorium and pushed them up against the front apron of the stage. The graduates were to descend from the stage down the roll-away stairs after receiving their diplomas. My mother took one look at the stairs, put down her broom and went home.

My grandmother had arranged for a gala in my mother's honor for that night, following the graduation. She'd invited every relative to the ceremony, made her daughter's graduation dress by hand and had the food and ice for the drinks already delivered to the house. But my mother refused to go to her graduation. She feared the steps would roll away from the stage just as she was descending to the audience. "You never know what might happen!" she cried to my incredulous grandmother. "What if I fell in front of all those people? What would they think? And Dad would be so upset if I got hurt!"

My grandmother argued fiercely with her. "Why would they roll away from you and not anyone else? Do you think you are the only person in the universe? What do you care what people think?" But she could not move her. My mother never graduated with her class, never wore the dress and never had the party. That night she stayed home in her bed. My grandfather supported her decision. My grandmother never understood why.

Several weeks later, my mother went to Coney Island amusement park with some friends. She tried to talk them into riding the Cyclone with her, the world's highest and fastest roller coaster, hurtling its passengers down the terrific inclines at speeds of eighty miles an hour. No one would get on with her but she didn't care. She climbed into the lead car alone, buckled herself in, and rode by herself in the front of the line of flimsy little cars as it inched its way, creaking and groaning, to the very top of the roller coaster. There she sat in the lead car as it hung for several seconds at the edge of the almost-vertical incline.

My mother looked down through the soft summer night at the thousands of twinkling white lights of the boardwalk far below. Perched high above the crowds, she felt safe because she knew that no one she valued could see her. She saw the crowds thronging the boardwalk and the game booths and penny arcades, the hot dog stands and souvenir shops. She saw the long strip of beach that ran next to the boardwalk and the dark, vast ocean beyond. But she didn't hear the roar of the waves. She heard only the faint, tinny music of the hurdy-gurdies and the carousel below. Whatever happened to her now was out of her control. Someone else was in charge of her destiny and she felt even more protected, excited. Someone else would have to take care of her. Her security rested on someone, anyone, else being in control.

She clutched the handrail as the car began to gather speed and then she screamed with delight as it hurtled downward to the bottom of the track, then up and then plunged down again with such terrific force that the new, gold wristwatch, a graduation present from her godmother that was to have been presented to her at her graduation gala, flew off her arm and was lost.

My grandmother never understood her younger daughter. My grandmother, Emily Ryan, was a big, regal-looking woman with a cloud of dark hair and brilliant blue eyes, and she was thirty-two years old that Sunday morning when she met my grandfather in the choir loft of Saint Agnes church. She was a strong-willed, sophisticated Englishwoman who had a successful career and was already an independent businesswoman, a dressmaker who had made Eleanor

Roosevelt's wedding dress and was much in demand to make dresses for other ladies of New York society.

She loved music, and she delighted in company. She insisted on having a piano in the house so she could play at the parties that she loved to give for her many friends and relatives. Her husband, much more "retiring" as she used to say, delighted in her enormous generosity and energy. He listened raptly when she played the piano, but sometimes when her playing was especially spirited he would say laughingly, "Play, Em! Don't pound!"

She made bathtub gin for Orange Blossom drinks to serve to the ladies of her bridge club, which met every Tuesday afternoon at the house on Ithaca Street. While her husband, Inspector Ryan, was leading raids on speakeasies over in Manhattan, his children were up in the bathroom of his house on Long Island scouring the bathtub free of any trace of gin before he got home.

The ladies always sat down around the dining room table for their bridge game. Over the table hung a chandelier of Waterford crystal, my grandmother's pride and joy. One Tuesday afternoon after the children finished scouring out the tub, they raced around the upstairs hall, laughing and chasing each other in and out of the bedrooms. My mother ran into her bedroom, jumped across the bed and ran to the door on the other side of the room. Her older brother, bigger and heavier than she, ran after her and jumped on the bed. The wooden bed cracked under his weight and he and the mattress slammed to the floor, directly over the dining room ceiling.

Downstairs were the ladies, deep into their bridge game and Orange Blossoms. The chandelier fell from the ceiling and smashed across the top of the dining room table, sending bits of splintered glass skittering across the table top like hailstones from a sudden, violent storm. The ladies sat, unhurt but stupefied, gaping at the glittering mess. After a long moment, my grandmother rose from the table. In a voice of deep and imperious calm, she called for her children.

"Here! You!"

"Who?" came several small voices from above.

"All!" said my grandmother.

All five trooped down the stairs and gathered silently around their mother.

"Who is responsible for this?"

"What?" said several of the children, their eyes fixed on the smashed glass and the staring women.

"I am," said my mother and my uncle, together.

"Go up and go into your rooms for the rest of the day. No supper. I will speak with both of you later," said my grandmother.

"Very well," said the two, and they went upstairs as they had been told. My mother often recounted that story. "No matter what," she would say. "Tell the truth." What did it matter that my grandmother had spent the morning making illegal gin? If someone had asked her she would have said, "Of course I did."

I could still see my grandmother at seventy years old, her head high and her cloud of white hair visible above the crowd of other pedestrians, striding alone down Ithaca Street to Roosevelt Avenue where she took the elevated train over to Brooklyn to Ebbett's Field to watch her beloved Dodgers play ball. She refused to miss an afternoon home-game. When her children were younger she would leave instructions: dinner (and dessert) were to be ready when she got home. "Natalie, bake your lemon meringue pie. Emily, you make the chicken and broccoli casserole. Tom, watch your little sisters. Peggy and Lucille, mind your brother." Her husband did not like her to go alone over to Brooklyn.

"Em, I wish you would not go unescorted. There are all those men! Think of what might happen! What will people think?" But she went anyway. On her way out the door she would say, "Why do you worry about what might happen? Of course I'm going! I'm in charge. I can take care of myself!"

Why didn't I inherit my Grandmother's spirit? Why, instead, did I learn to feel as helpless as my grandfather?

Why did the unexpected overcome them? Because both men viewed themselves as helpless, powerless in a world in which anything "might" happen. Now I knew that the men hadn't been defeated by those events. My grandfathers were victims of themselves, of their own fearful perceptions. And this is exactly why I'm fearful, I thought, lying in my hospital bed. I have learned to feel helpless. Like my parents, I have learned to believe that I have no control.

And yet my parents packed our belongings, put everything they owned into storage and set out for what they thought was a new future. My mother and father were excited about their trip together across the country. Neither one had ever been away from New York. They'd met at a high school dance in Queens when both were seniors. My father was four years older than all the senior boys. He'd had to leave high school at seventeen to support his widowed mother and couldn't return to finish his senior year until he was twenty-one. My mother was attracted to him immediately because he was older. She saw the gentle care he took of his mother, and she assumed he would take the same care of her. They'd been married only a year before I was born and then had come the fright of six years of war. Was this journey their way of overcoming the fears that had always haunted them? Might this new adventure lead to a life they could finally control?

We left for California in late June 1948. We drove for almost two weeks. My brother and I sat in the back of the new car, and my little sister rode with my mother in front. We drove through New Jersey and then Ohio, then Indiana and across Missouri and into Oklahoma. The country was becoming strange to me, a sheltered child used to leafy suburbs and city streets. We drove through vast, empty stretches of land and along dark, empty roads at night. There was only blackness until in the distance we saw the red or blue glare of neon lights on the horizon that signaled the next town and the next motel where we would stop for the night. One night outside of Tulsa, my parents found a cafeteria-style restaurant next to the motel. After dinner, I had a bowl of red Jell-O for dessert. As soon as I finished it, I felt horribly sick to my stomach. My mother took me downstairs to a restroom where she waited with me, thinking I would throw up my entire dinner, but I didn't. Instead I was seized with horrible cramps that only lessened after she insisted that we would rest for the night and not leave in the morning until I felt better.

We had been driving for days, and we were still very far from California. What if I delayed the trip because I felt sick? What if they had to keep stopping along the way just because of me? My mother and father were having such a good time. They'd looked forward to this trip for so long. I was terrified of being sick to my stomach, not just in their new car, but in a strange place. I tried not to think about the cramps, but every afternoon, just before we were to stop for the night, they would overcome me again. I'd brought my books with me, *Heidi,* the *Bobbsey Twins, The Five Little Peppers and How They Grew,* and I tried to lose myself in reading. I said nothing, fearing my father's patience would snap. I was silent while they drove. After all, they were driving thousands of miles alone across unknown country with three little children. But my father had been strangely calm and quiet as we drove, and many times during the trip he called out to me in the back seat to look at this sight or another.

"Yes, I see that, Daddy!"

My brother stared out the window silently. He didn't speak at all. When he was tired he would lean close against me and fall asleep.

Near Gallup, New Mexico, my father stopped at a gas station to double check the radiator and the oil in the car. My mother brought my little sister into the gas station to go to the bathroom. My brother and I got out of the car and went over to sit at an old picnic table that was set up by the side of the road. We wore our summer clothes in the dry desert heat. I had on a short sundress and sandals. I over-heard the mechanic talking to my father.

"That your little girl?" he asked my father.

"Yes," said my father.

"She's real pretty," said the man.

"Thank you," my father said.

"But she looks like a spider. I ain't never seen such long arms and legs."

I saw my father turn his head and look at me.

"She don't smile much," said the man.

We reached Flagstaff, Arizona, the next day. My stomach cramps were so painful that I lay curled up in the back seat. My brother sat close to me and quietly stroked my hair. Neither of us spoke. My mother kept looking anxiously into the back seat.

"I wish you would find a hospital," she said to my father.

The hospital was a low, flat building, painted white and sur-rounded by tall fir trees. It seemed to dazzle in the sun. The emer-gency room had venetian blinds drawn against the afternoon sun. The doctor was a young man with black hair and dark eyes. He spoke very softly to me as he pressed his hands against my stomach. Then he went to the door and called my parents into the room.

"There's nothing physically wrong with your daughter," he said. "But she's very afraid of making you upset." He looked at my father. "She doesn't want to say that she misses her home. She doesn't know where you're taking her."

We arrived in Santa Monica in time for the opening of the school year and moved into Mr. and Mrs. Zavitkovsy's garage. My father spent the days looking for work, and my mother stayed in the garage with my little sister, trying to make it a home. I was enrolled in the third grade at the nearby Catholic school. My brother entered the first grade. He hated the school. He stayed to himself in the class-room, and when the nun approached him to join the others he screamed. He cried so uncontrollably that I would be called from the third-grade classroom many times to take him home.

My classmates dressed up after school when they went out to play. The girls changed from their school uniforms into pink, organdy dresses and shiny, white patent-leather shoes and white socks with lacy trim. They wore satin ribbons in their long, blonde hair. The boys wore new blue jeans and crisp, plaid shirts and cowboy boots. They wore cowboy hats, like Roy Rogers, on top of their blonde hair. Everyone, everywhere you looked, was blonde. The boys and girls said they might be "discovered" by some movie director in jodhpurs and riding boots. I thought it was odd that they never looked at you when they talked to you, but somewhere over your shoulder, as if expecting someone to appear out of nowhere and whisk them off to stardom in the movies.

The Christmas Eve that we spent in California was surreal, like a nightmare. As the day went on, the weather grew balmier, sunnier. People talked of spending the holiday at the beach. Exotic flowers bloomed everywhere and palm trees swayed in the gentle ocean breeze. That evening at dinner, my brother, who was five, and my sister, just three, wondered how Santa Claus could come without any snow for his sled and reindeer.

"Oh," laughed Mr. Zavitkovsky. "He's coming right now! Look!"

We all went outside and looked up into the warm night sky. As if on cue, we heard the sound of an approaching helicopter. The clumsy thing whirled and clanked its way toward us, over the palm trees. There, in the open side door was a person dressed as Santa Claus. "Merry Christmas!" he screamed through a megaphone.

We hated it. We all hated it. We left two weeks later, to drive back to New York in early January 1948. I was not sick once. We arrived in a blizzard that struck just as we entered New Jersey. We had to spend one last night in a motel, but we didn't mind. We were thrilled just to see the snow.

We spent the next several weeks with my Grandmother Ryan in her house on Ithaca Street, and a short time later my father got a job in Connecticut as the advertising manager for the Bridgeport Brass Company. In Fairfield, he rented an old white house with steeply sloping gables at the end of a small street called Benson Place. Maple trees lined both sides of the street. The trees met and formed a canopy of bare, dark red branches over the street. At the end of the street was a gate that led to a sandy path through a wide salt marsh and then to a beach on Long Island Sound. The first night that we lived there, I stood at the window of the new bedroom I shared with my little sister. I heard the faint, clanging noise of buoy bells far out in the Sound. I listened to the sounds of new life in the marsh that surrounded us: the tiny, peeping cries of baby frogs and the rustle of the soft spring wind as it brushed through the tall reeds and rushes. I watched the wind move the bare branches of the maple trees just outside the window. The branches swayed and caught together and then the wind pulled them gently away from each other and then moved them back until they caught again. It seemed a place of safety for us. Maybe there was no longer any reason for my parents to be fearful. Maybe now they could be happy. I wondered at the silence and the peace of this place we had finally come to. I wondered if it would last. I was ten years old.

ᘓᘓᘓᘓᘓᘓ

Sometime later in the night the anesthesiologist woke me. He was a small, dark man with gray hair who sat down in the chair next to my bed. He sat quietly in the semidarkness as if exhausted, his legs stretched out in front of him and his hands clasped loosely in his lap. He still wore light blue scrubs and a small, light blue cap on his head.

The cap was pushed far back on his head like a yarmulke.

"How are you?" he asked. He had an accent that I couldn't place. Czech? Austrian?

"Fine," I said. I was only half-awake. "How are you?"

"Good."

"What country are you from?" I asked.

"Israel," he said. "Why do you want to know?"

"You sound different."

"Oh," he said. "You're funny. Not many patients tell me I sound different."

"You look very tired," I said.

"They don't tell me that either," he said. "It's usually the other way around."

"Please be sure I wake up."

"You may count on it," he said.

He stayed for a minute sitting there, smiling at me from his chair as if I was some odd, unexpected character he hadn't expected to meet there at night in the hospital.

"Good night," he said, getting up. "I'll see you in the morning." He laid his hand on my foot at the bottom of the bed. "Thank you for thinking of me," he said, and went out.

Now I knew that in the morning my breast would be cut off. I wondered what they would do with it. There is something uncertain, something strange and unfinished, about an amputation. I could imagine how my body would look without my breast. But my poor breast! What would become of it? What would become of me? What could I do about any of the things that were about to happen to me? "Fear leads toward death," wrote Seneca. "Courage leads to the stars." "My own fear will kill me, like my grandfathers," I said out loud. "Unless I understand it. Then I can control it." I knew I had to break the helpless cycle. I had to begin to see this disease as a battle I could win. If I could meet it with a feeling of control and hope I could beat it. Others had done it. Why couldn't I? I closed my eyes and made myself imagine the weak cancer cells. "Damn you all," I said out loud. "I'm so sick of weakness. I will be in control. Get out."

CHAPTER SIX

The Mastectomy: Day Two

I woke sometime before dawn on the morning of my operation not knowing where I was. Confused, I stared around the room. Suddenly, with a shock, I remembered. I flung the bedcovers off, got out of the bed and ran out, breathless, into the hall. There was the night nurse, just coming toward me. "Hey," she said. "You're supposed to be in bed. You're due in the OR in a few minutes."

"I'm scared," I said.

"I know," she said, "but I brought something to calm you down. Get back in bed and roll over." I did as I was told and she administered a stinging injection into my backside.

"Oh, my God!" I gasped. "What is that?"

"Muscle relaxer," she said, briskly. "You'll feel wonderful in less than a minute."

Even as she said the words, a warm and peaceful sensation flooded through me. I smiled up at her happily. An orderly appeared next to my bed, an older black man with a thin, gray moustache. I felt myself being lifted out of the bed and onto a gurney, and then the orderly pushed me out into the hall and down a long corridor. As he pushed me, I gazed at the lights of the hallway as they flashed by above me. I heard snatches of conversation as I rolled along. The orderly stopped at the elevator, and when the door opened, he swung the gurney around and pushed me through the door. I saw faces, as if disembodied, looking down at me as I lay there.

The elevator door opened and the orderly rolled my gurney into a long dim hallway outside the operating rooms. I could see long rows of other gurneys waiting, lined up against the walls, the patients hidden under mounds of bedding. I saw someone dressed in light blue scrubs standing between the gurneys as if waiting for someone. It was Dr. McCullough. As soon as he saw me, he came over to me. He walked along with me as I rolled into the operating room.

"I just wanted to tell you that I'll take good care of you. Everything will be fine," he said. "I'll see you a little later."

Even in my dreamy state I knew he'd been waiting for me.

"Thank you," I said. But I thought that I hadn't thanked him enough.

In the operating room, bright lights shone on gleaming tile walls and stainless steel countertops. Nurses in light blue scrubs and white, gauzy hats that looked like oversized shower caps bustled about. Two of them lifted me quickly up off my gurney and onto the operating table. The top of it was shockingly cold. It was so narrow that I suddenly felt as though I would fall off. My hands clutched at the sides of it. I stared up. Above the operating table a huge, glaring, round light shone directly down on me. Suddenly the drowsy feeling I'd had was gone. "Wait!" I thought. "Not yet! Wait!" I thought of getting up, off the operating table, but I realized I couldn't move my legs. They felt heavy, weighted down. I began to tremble violently. I tried to remember what I'd read. Take control of the smallest thing first. Be calm.

"I'm very cold," I said to the nurse who was standing over me. "Would you please cover me with something?"

"Sure," she said, and put a warm blanket over me.

"We meet again," said a voice over my left shoulder.

The anesthesiologist came around the operating table and smiled down at me. He looked rested. He laid his hand gently on my arm.

"Hello," he said in his faint accent. "I told you I'd take care of you."

"Please be sure I wake up," I said again.

"Don't worry," he said. "Can you count backward from ten?"

"Yes," I said. "Why would I want to do that?"

"Because I'll know you're asleep when you stop counting. You'll be asleep before you get to one."

"Oh, okay," I said. "Ten. Nine." Then I fell asleep.

❦❦❦

I woke in the afternoon with the same, pleasant, drowsy feeling I'd had in the early morning. Rita and another younger nurse were busy arranging blankets around me. The younger one put a pillow under my right elbow. I was vaguely aware of a big, bulky mound of bandages on top of the right side of my chest but I couldn't feel any pain there.

"Pat asked me to tell you that he's outside," said Rita. "Would you like him to come in?"

"I probably don't look so hot," I said.

"He's been waiting to see you for hours," she said. "I don't think he'll care how you look."

She went over to the door and nodded to someone out in the hall. Pat came into the room with a single red rose in his hand. He leaned over and kissed me on my forehead. His face was strange, drawn, and he had dark circles under his eyes. He seemed hesitant, cautious, as if he was frightened of me for some reason.

"I love you," he said. "I'll call you tonight."

He laid the rose and a small blue card next to me on the bed and left.

"Is that your husband?" asked the younger nurse.

"No," I said.

"He's been here since eleven this morning," she said. "We took turns bringing him coffee."

"We got a little concerned about him," said Rita.

"Why?" I said.

The younger nurse looked down. I could see that she had tears in her eyes.

"What happened?" I said.

"He was so worried about you," said the younger nurse. "When I went into the waiting room, he was standing by himself over in the corner of the room and he was crying. It was hard to see him so upset . . . a big man like that standing there with his shoulders shaking, holding that red rose in his hands." She looked at me. "I hope someone loves me like that some day."

I tried to reach for the card he had left on the bed but I couldn't move my right arm. The nurse put it in my left hand. On it he'd written, "Hurry! We have a life to live! I love you."

෯෯෯෯

I'd met Pat in the summer of 1979, just a few months before I began to teach at Choate. I was having dinner with Tim, an old friend, at the only restaurant on the main street in the center of Fairfield, Connecticut, where I grew up. Pat was at the bar. I knew of him . . . he was a writer, and he had gone to the local Catholic university with my former husband. Pat and I had never met, which was unusual because we had grown up in the same small town and knew many of the same people. Tim invited him over to join us for a drink. Pat told me he had seen me often through the years. He knew about my divorce.

He was a big man, muscular, broad-shouldered. He had black curly hair, deep brown eyes, a full-lipped mouth and the dark stubble of a beard. He was gracious but removed. There were little laugh creases around his eyes, but he didn't laugh often, or easily. He was thirty-seven that summer, but he looked much older, weary, preoccupied, as if absorbed in some sad problem known only to himself. He didn't stay long at our table. He excused himself abruptly and left the restaurant. He was married, Tim said, with children and a hopelessly dependent wife. I watched him walk slowly, head down, until he reached his car parked under the trees across the street from the restaurant. Then I saw him turn and glance back, squinting as if to see more clearly through the glass window, at me, as I sat staring out at him.

Several weeks later he called me. He asked if I would meet him at the beach near my father's house where I was staying before my move with Annie to Choate. I didn't know why he called me or wanted to see me, and I didn't even consider that I was meeting a married man. For some reason that I didn't understand, I met him that afternoon on the beach.

We talked that day about books we liked, people we knew, about our children and then we talked about my divorce. He seemed to understand me when I told him about the loneliness of my failed marriage, but at first he said nothing. It surprised us both when we noticed that it was late afternoon, the beach was deserted and that we had spent hours talking.

Pat was the only son of hot-tempered Italian parents. He'd spent the early part of his childhood hearing violent arguments between his father, a professional gambler, and his mother, a small, dark, ferocious woman who had no patience with her husband's losses. Pat's father loved gambling, but when he lost, the house itself was in peril because he lost the money to pay the mortgage. "But I don't dwell on my losses!" screamed his father. "No! I forget them! That's the past! I concentrate on the next game!" This, of course, enraged his wife. "Nothing simmered in our house," Pat told me. "I never knew when they would explode at each other."

He hated the volatile atmosphere of the house and freed himself from its chaos by escaping to the town baseball field where he learned to pitch. By the time he was ten he was a prodigy. When he graduated from the local Catholic prep school, in 1959, he was given a fifty-thousand-dollar bonus by the Milwaukee Braves. He bought his parents their house—one way of ending some of their violent arguments. Then he left home to pitch in the minor leagues.

But in spite of his astonishing talent, he failed to make the major leagues. Three years after he left home as a high school sensation, he was released from the minor leagues and returned to Fairfield, bitter, angry and confused. He was twenty-one.

He'd married his high school sweetheart, a beautiful blonde girl, who was sweet, passive and comforting. He went back to college, the local Catholic university, and took two or three part-time jobs to support his growing family. But he always thought of himself as a baseball pitcher and the loss of his talent haunted him. The more he tried to understand the cause of his failure, the more confused he became.

One of the part-time jobs he had at night was for the Bridgeport Post, the area newspaper. He wrote the tiny headlines for the small, two-paragraph high school sports articles that appeared at the bottom of the sports section. He liked the order his headlines imposed on the paragraphs. He discovered that when he imposed order on his thoughts, as he did on his headlines, he could make sense of reality.

Soon, he began to write the sports articles and then, gradually, he began to write about himself. Through his writing, he came to understand his failure. In his book, A *False Spring*, he remembered himself as a young pitcher, standing on the mound in such total control of the game and the batters who faced him that instead of concentrating on his next pitch, his thoughts would leap ahead to his next success, and then the next, until he found himself losing first the game, then his temper, then his career, and finally, his innocence. The game and the order he tried to impose on it hadn't failed him. He'd lost control of himself.

So he taught himself to control his thoughts and reactions. The impulsive man became careful and patient. The control he gained over himself and his thoughts freed him from his anxiety, fear and confusion. He saw his writing as a way of ordering his thoughts so as to understand reality. He saw it as a way he could discover the truth, which he prized above all. However, the truth was, that no matter what order he tried to maintain, the unexpected would happen. But he wanted to be prepared. He didn't want to be powerless. He tried to be in control.

And then he lost his marriage. He told me about the emptiness of it. His wife was a soft, pale, reserved woman who, after the birth of their youngest child, refused to have sex with him. So he lost himself in his writing. He began to take Valium to ease the unexplained headaches he suffered. After he spent his days writing and taking his wife, who didn't drive, to the grocery store and his children to and from school, he fell asleep early on the living room sofa while his wife and children watched television. When they went to bed he stayed downstairs and slept by himself on the sofa.

If his wife knew about his desolation, she said nothing. That was his sorrow. He began to go out at night rather than spend lonely hours downstairs by himself. Soon he found solace in other women and in the Valium, which he began to wash down with vodka. He mourned his lost marriage and reviled himself as the reason for its failure. His wife did nothing to assuage his guilt and loneliness. She became more distant and self-absorbed. If she knew about the other women, she said nothing. She supported him in his work and kept the house running smoothly so he could write upstairs in his attic room. He was committed to taking care of his children and of his wife. But if he left her, he believed, his house and family would fall apart. So he persevered. When I met him, he had not slept with her for ten years. He was tired, sad, alone. Then he fell in love with me.

He called me often after that summer day we spent talking on the beach. He seemed eager to share something he'd written or ask what I thought about a movie that had just come out. I found myself waiting to hear from him so I could tell him about one of the English courses I was preparing to teach in the fall or ask him what he thought about my youngest daughter's fears about moving to a new town and a new school. But I didn't see him again until one afternoon almost at the end of the summer. He knew I was moving soon, up to Choate. He wondered if I would meet him later that night for a drink at the restaurant in town to say good-bye. I was surprised at myself . . . at how much I looked forward to seeing him. I didn't realize then that I was falling in love with him. That night he told me that he had tried not to see me before I moved away from town. He told me that he'd gone to the beach hoping to see me but left whenever he did see me walking down the path from my father's house.

We left the restaurant and walked across the street to where our cars were parked under the trees. As I turned to open the door of my car he touched my arm. "Don't go yet," he said softly. He had a small office on the top floor of one of the old houses that lined the main street of the town. We turned and walked together along the main street toward the house. We went in and without speaking climbed the stairs to the third floor. He hesitated for a moment in the hall before he opened the door to his office. He turned to look at me. "Are you sure?" he asked.

"Yes," I said. "I'm sure."

We lay down on the floor of his office and held each other. No one had ever held me as tenderly as he did. And then we began, slowly, to make love. Later, he lay next to me, looking down at me.

"I love you," he said.

He said it so sadly that I thought he had said something else. In the dark shadows of his office, I couldn't see his face.

"What?" I said.

"I love you," he said, and he shook his head and sighed.

Two months later, he felt the lump on my breast. He didn't tell me then that after I left him that night, to drive back to Wallingford, he spent the night without sleeping, afraid that I would be taken away from him. That he couldn't control what had happened to me. And he was afraid. I didn't tell him what I was thinking. That this was the calamity I had dreaded but half-expected. Who was I to think I had a future?

∾∾∾∾∾

Much later that night, the woman whose bed was next to mine returned from the operating room. The night nurse asked her several times if there was anything she wanted, anything she needed. But the woman made no response. Her phone rang several times, but she didn't answer it. She lay there, silent, motionless, in the dark. *Why does she shut herself off?* I wondered. It occurred to me that we're not required to confront our fears alone. The support of others is there if we aren't too desolate to accept it.

Once, I had been desolate. I remembered my loneliness in the years before this day. I'd never told anyone of my fears or sorrows, my losses or confusion. I didn't think that I could ask for anything for myself—even in my prayers. Because I was silent, I had increased the weight of my own suffering. But that morning, when I was afraid on the operating table, as a way of controlling my fear, I'd asked the nurse for a blanket. I realized that I'd done something profoundly important. I had asked for help.

I thought about the kindness of everyone I'd met that day. I was glad I'd accepted the care each person offered. I touched the card Pat left me. "Hurry! We have a life to live! I love you." Once, I feared no man could ever love me, especially as a single woman, disfigured, with one breast. I wondered if I could resolve to get well again if Pat were not in my life. *Yes,* I thought. *I have to try. This is what I have to do for myself. What a remarkable day I've had,* I thought. *Maybe I can be in control. Can this be the first day of my new life? How I want to live! I can't wait for tomorrow!*

CHAPTER SEVEN

The Hemorrhage: Day Three

The next morning, I woke to the voice of a nurse's aide standing by the side of my bed with a breakfast tray. She helped me gently out of bed into a chair and put the tray in my lap. I looked out the window at a brilliant, cloudless blue sky and then suddenly fell asleep, face down, into the bowl of Kellogg's Special-K on the tray. The loud, frightened voice of the aide woke me as she wiped the milk and cereal out of my eyes and nose. I kept nodding lazily away to sleep in my chair, vaguely aware that Rita and another nurse had rushed into the room. They lifted me out of the chair and back onto my bed. Rita rolled me over on my left side and looked, for some reason, at my back.

"Get a gurney!" she said. "Quick!" The other nurse ran to the door and called loudly to someone in the hall. "Get Dr. McCullough! He's on his way to the game!"

What game? I thought. "Ah," I said to myself. "Harvard, Yale." I wondered why everyone around me was screaming.

I felt myself lifted onto a gurney and something very cold go into my left arm and then into my shoulder. I looked up into the frightened face of the nurse and saw that she kept slapping a still frozen packet of blood that hung on a hanger next to my head. I watched the dark red pouch dance crazily up and down on its hanger. I tried to stay awake, to concentrate on the anxious face of the nurse who was bending over me, but the urge to sleep was overwhelming.

I woke later, in the operating room, to the sound of someone moaning. Dr. McCullough was standing next to me, once again in his blue scrubs. He was talking over me to another doctor on my left side.

"Who is that crying?" I asked.

"That was you," he said. "But you're awake now."

"What happened?" I said.

"You had a hemorrhage," he said.

In the recovery room, I struggled to open my eyes. I felt someone gently stroking my hair.

"Who is that?" I asked.

"It's John," said a voice. "Monica's husband." He came around to where I could see him.

"You had a rough day," he said. "We almost lost you."

"Yeah," I said. "But I'm still here."

"Good," he said, laughing. "But Pat is very worried. Let me have someone call him and tell him you're okay."

"Thank you," I said. "Thank you all for everything."

It's true that some illnesses might overcome even the most indomitable spirit, like bombs really falling, or like the hemorrhage I had. But I'd survived that. I had a second chance. I didn't know then that the days I spent in the hospital because of that hemorrhage would be the beginning of my new life. That night I was still too weak to get my body out of bed, but I did my visualizations. Always after those times of mental imagery and concentration on making myself well again, I felt completely calm, strong and in control. I used those times to remember . . . to go back again to my childhood. I was learning that remembering is a way of healing. Why was I afraid to think of myself first when I was young? When did that lesson begin?

ᐯᐯᐯᐯᐯ

The first tiny red buds of spring had just appeared on the maple trees when we moved to Fairfield, Connecticut, a town on the southeastern coast of Long Island Sound just across from Long Island, New York. Puritans left the Plymouth colony in Massachusetts, moved southwest down the Atlantic coast into Connecticut and settled the town in 1639. The lands had been the home of the Pequot Nation, a fierce tribe of Native Americans who fought the Puritans in vain to keep their homes and their heritage. One such Puritan was a Captain John Underhill who attacked a Pequot village and destroyed it. He burned the Pequot homes with their families still inside. Of the four hundred Pequot in that village, five survived the slaughter. After the attack Underhill quoted from the Bible . . . and then wrote a letter explaining his actions. "Sometimes the Scripture says that women and children must perish with their parents. We had sufficient light from the word of God for our proceedings." By 1637, the Pequot were vanquished, and the Puritans began to settle their lands in Connecticut in earnest. Fairfield was settled in 1639; in the next year, 1640, the town became part of the New Haven Colony, established by a Puritan minister named John Davenport. The laws that governed Fairfield then were even more rigid than those of the rest of Connecticut. Strict rules controlled all aspects of moral and religious life. Puritans had overwhelmed the free Pequot, slaughtered their women and children, taken their lands, and annihilated their civilization and heritage in order to provide a place where God's laws would be followed to the letter. God's mercy and love would shine on the Puritans as long as they destroyed any threat to their beliefs.

When we moved there in 1948, Fairfield was a prim, straitlaced New England town of old white colonial houses, spacious lawns and towering trees. The Boston Post Road, the old highway that connected Boston to New York City in the early colonial days, divided the town and had become Fairfield's main street. On the west side of the Post Road, as we called it, the land sloped up toward the old farms of Greenfield Hill, where farmers, as they grew more prosperous, acquired bigger tracts of land and built more spacious homes that looked out from the Hill over the town to the Sound beyond.

On the east side of the road, the beach side next to the Sound where we lived, stately old colonial houses still lined the old streets, named for some of the founding fathers of the town: Burr, Rowland, Penfield, Benson. There were also the remnants of estates that had once stretched unbroken to the white sands of the beach. In the fronts of the houses were still the small blocks of gray stone with iron rings set in that were used to tie the reins of the horses that once pulled carriages along the road the century before. Then, a lady could alight from her carriage onto the stone and be helped to the ground by a liveried manservant.

The borders of old formal gardens remained, with the foundations of reflecting pools still intact. There were parts of old bridle paths that led from the houses through the marsh to the beach. These were the homes and estates that had once belonged to the colonists loyal to the British crown during the Revolutionary War. Everything else had been torched, burned to the ground by the British redcoats when they sailed up Long Island Sound, landed on Fairfield beach, marched down our road, shot any dissenters and destroyed the houses of those who were suspected to be revolutionaries. Only the field-stone foundations of these houses remained.

By 1948 there were no more revolutionaries. It seemed as if the ghosts of the British redcoats and the old Puritans were marching through the town together. "Conform or perish!"

When I was a young girl growing up there in the 1950s, the strict, old Puritan ethic had returned. It was as if dour, old Parson Davenport had come back in his dusty, black-frocked coat and given the present inhabitants a stern warning: that the heady freedom gained during the Revolution was embarrassing . . . wrong somehow. It was a liberation that should have been savored briefly, if at all. And in the Fairfield of 1950, freedom was a fearsome, uncertain thing. What would you do with it? Fairfield was a place where you wore what everyone else wore, behaved the way everyone else did and thought the way everyone else thought. In those days, in the 1950s, as it was in most of America, you were expected to conform, fit in. In Fairfield in those years, any independent idea or action was looked upon with suspicion and a particular kind of New England disdain.

But the strict traditions of the town gave my mother and father a sense of great comfort and security. My parents didn't like change. They were afraid of it. They'd always been afraid of "what might happen." They wanted someone else to be in charge, to tell them what to do. They wanted to be protected, controlled, to do what everyone else was doing. They felt secure within the rigid doctrines and laws of the Catholic Church. They felt safe watched over by the priests of our parish, in the traditional, old New England town, in our little house surrounded and protected by the marsh. But when I was a young girl, I was free there . . . for a time.

When we first walked in to the house on Benson Place, there was already a small stack of wood piled neatly next to the fireplace in the living room. At the back of the living room was a narrow stairway that led to the hall and three bedrooms above. A sun porch with a long row of windows was to the left, off the living room. The windows faced out to the side lawn and the gate at the end of the street that opened onto the marsh. To the right of the living room was the dining room, and beyond that in the back of the house was a large kitchen. The kitchen windows looked out over the back-yard, where a thin strip of lawn met the tall reeds and bulrushes of the marsh.

Upstairs, my little sister and I had one of the bedrooms that faced the street with its row of maple trees. My Grandmother Ryan had given us her big old four-poster bed and a bureau that had been my Aunt Lucille's. Our room had a long closet and a tiny window at the end of the room that looked out over the side yard to the marsh and the Sound beyond. I could stand at the window in the morning and watch the sun as it rose and glistened on the waters of the Sound. From that window, I watched the color of the marsh grasses and bul-rushes change with the seasons from pale silver green in spring, to rich, deep green in summer, then, as autumn came, to a soft buff then silvery gray again with the winter.

I could never stay in the house for long. The scent of rain coming in the warm afternoons, the soft rustle of the new leaves of the maple trees, the sharp, salt smell that rose from the marsh on the first warm, humid nights, the sound of the foghorn from the end of Penfield Reef, brought me either out of the house or to an open window.

A wide, white sandy path cut through the marsh to the beach. One afternoon, just after we moved in, I left the path and set out across the marsh. As I brushed through the tall reeds and new grasses, I came to a sudden clearing. An old bridle path of worn, flat fieldstones ran between two rows of aged apple trees to the beach. The trees were twisted and stunted but heavy with masses of pale, pink bloom. As I started down the path under the trees, an anxious, squawking noise came from the tree just above me. A mother bird flapped and hopped nervously about on one of the upper branches. I climbed into the tree and saw that she'd built a nest, almost hidden in the crook of two branches. I climbed further up in the tree to look inside it. There in the small, deep circle of her nest lay three small, pale blue eggs. I had never seen anything so perfect, so alone, so beautiful. The mother's cries grew louder and more frantic, and she began to make swooping dives at my head. "Don't worry," I said to her. "I won't ever touch them," and I climbed down.

I went back after school every day and climbed into the tree to see the eggs. The mother grew used to me, but I stayed for only seconds and climbed down again, not wanting to frighten her. One day, as I approached the tree I heard faint cheeping sounds coming from the nest above. I climbed up anxiously, afraid something might have happened to the mother. There in the nest was a huddle of naked, soft pink flesh. As I looked, three baby birds picked up wobbly heads from the tender, pink mass. Their eyes were squeezed tightly shut and their heads swayed about, far too big for their tiny bodies. Suddenly they opened their yellow beaks! Their mouths were wide, gaping, eager, as if expecting something. From me! What could I give them?! I stared, transfixed, breathless, until I saw the mother bird circle the tree. She hopped lightly onto one of the upper branches and regarded me with beady, black eyes. "I told you I wouldn't touch them," I said to her. "You know what to do." In the next days, I couldn't wait for school to end in the afternoon. I sat as if imprisoned at my desk and stole glances at the clock as the hour hand moved slowly to three. Every stop on the school bus route so frustrated me that I wanted to get out and run home. I rushed into the house, changed out of my school uniform, put on my jeans, and ran furiously over to the orchard. Over the next few weeks, the babies' skinny bodies grew bigger and plumper and fit the size of their heads. Soft white down appeared on their little bodies, followed soon after by sleek, brown feathers. I was convinced they knew me. And the mother bird, who had been so anxious when I'd first discovered her new nest, now seemed tranquil and content when I came to visit her little ones. One day I ran all the way to the orchard without even changing my uniform. As usual, I approached the tree carefully so as not to frighten the mother, but there seemed to be a strange silence above. I climbed into the tree and looked into the nest. It was empty, deserted. There was nothing in it to show that my sweet little birds had even been there except several baby feathers of white down.

Later that spring my father came home from work carrying a cardboard box in his arms. He always walked the mile from the bus stop on the Boston Post Road down North Benson Road to our house at the end of Benson Place. He put the box down on the kitchen floor.

"This is for you, Susan," he said.

I knelt down and looked inside the box. A small black puppy sat in the bottom of the box, staring up at me with soulful brown eyes. I was overwhelmed at the sight of her. I picked her up out of the box and held her close to my face. She smelled of the same fresh, sweet scent I remembered when I had bent down to kiss my baby sister as I rocked her as an infant, years before. I burst into tears.

"I hope she makes you happy, Susan," my father said. "She's yours."

"Oh, thank you, Daddy!" I said. "How did you know I wanted her?"

"Your mother told me."

I called her Pepper, and I took her everywhere with me except to school. Because my mother wouldn't allow her to sleep in my bedroom she slept in the kitchen. She was overjoyed to see me every morning, as if I had been away from her for years. One day, when I was at school and she was about six months old, she slipped out of the backyard through a small hole in the wire fence that separated the yard from the marsh. My mother hadn't missed her. My dog didn't run to greet me after school when I came home into the kitchen. I looked frantically, all through the marsh along the old bridle path between the apple trees, up and down the beach. I was heartsick, terrified at the thought of what might have happened to her. When my father came home he went straight to the phone, waited for the party line to clear and called the dog pound to see if anyone had found her. He called several times. Night came, and no one had found her. Somehow I got through the next school day, rushed home from the school-bus stop and into the kitchen, hoping she would run to meet me. But she wasn't there. I was beyond tears. My father came home and called the *Bridgeport Post* newspaper and placed an ad under Lost and Found. We were just sitting down to dinner when the phone rang. My mother answered it.

"Oh, thank heaven," she said. "My daughter has been beside herself."

A woman across the marsh, on Beach Road, had found my dog. Pepper had wandered into her backyard and slept on her back porch all the night before. The woman had called the dog warden who gave her our phone number.

"I could tell she was very important to someone," the woman told my mother. "She's a sweet, loving little dog."

"Come on," said my father to me. "Let's get her."

"Thank you, Daddy," I said.

"I know how much you love her," he said. "I know she makes you very happy."

Later that night, before I went to bed, I went into the living room where my father was reading his newspaper.

"Thank you for helping me find my dog. I love you, Daddy."

"I love you, too. Now go to bed."

In summer, the first wind before a thunderstorm moved gently through the maple trees and touched the leaves. It lifted the silver undersides of the maple leaves up and turned them over, and they shimmered and quivered in anticipation of the rain to come. As the storm grew, the trees sighed and swayed and bent away from the wind, but then, as if unable to help themselves, they leaned forward again to meet it. In summer, we walked down the wide, white path through the marsh to the beach. In those days, the waters of Long Island Sound were clear as the air. We dove off the wooden raft that was anchored some yards out from the shore and swam underwater and picked up the pink and pale yellow shells that littered the white sand under the surface, and we held swimming races to see who swam the fastest or who could last the longest underwater without coming up for air, and we formed underwater circles with other children and stared googley-eyed at each other under the surface until one of us broke the clear underwater calm and laughed with a great burst of bubbles. Then we rose to the surface and floated on our backs and stared straight up at a sky that seemed limitless.

Some summer mornings, my brother and I took Pepper and walked through the marsh over to Ash Creek, a broad, deep channel that cut through the marsh and flowed into the Sound and where the local fishermen moored their small boats. We brought a metal bucket and a small net attached to the end of a long wooden pole, salvaged from one of my mother's old mops. We brought lengths of string and chunks of table scraps left over from dinner the night before. My brother and I sat at the end of the old wooden dock and tied the scraps onto the long lengths of string and dropped the scraps down into the water where they floated alluringly among the underwater pilings of the dock. We dropped the pole down quietly and watched as the net settled softly into the sand. Then we threw ourselves down on our stomachs on the dock and stared off the edge into the water and waited. Soon, a round, flat shape would emerge from between the pilings and a pair of pincer-like claws would slowly approach the scrap tied to the end of the string. We held our breath and watched, our eyes fixed on the two claws as they moved toward the scrap and then suddenly encircled it. We felt the sharp tug at the string and moved the net stealthily behind the crab and captured it. We pulled it up, its dusky blue shell now shining in the sunlight and its claws waving at us as if in a slow motion greeting. Pepper sat motionless on the dock, her brown eyes following as the crab waved its strange, thin blue arms above the rim of the pail like some small, exotic, sea dancer beckoning us all back into the sea. Hours later we went back home across the marsh, our metal pail full of blue crabs, their claws clanking and scratching against the sides. The first time we brought home a catch of blue crabs my mother screamed. She refused to touch them. She would not cook them, so we gave them to Mrs. Benway who lived up the street. My grandmother tried to explain to my mother that these were prized seafood and should be boiled with certain spices, but my mother never went anywhere near them. My brother and I caught them anyway and gave them to the families on our street who loved them.

In October, the leaves on the maple trees turned brilliant gold. The leaves glimmered in the dense, heavy fog that surrounded our house on those first chilly autumn mornings. On those mornings, my father got up early, before the rest of us were out of bed. He went down to the cellar and shoveled coal into the furnace, and the heat would come up in the house, hissing and clanking in the radiators. He always tried to keep the house warm for us. In the cold, bright afternoons, the smoke rose from those golden leaves as they burned in piles at the end of the driveways, curling up into the crisp air and hanging in a blue haze over the street.

Eight families lived on Benson Place. After dinner, we children cut cattails from the bulrushes in the marsh and poked them into the still-glowing embers of the fires. The ends of the cattails caught fire and smoked and gave off a pungent smell of slow-burning

brine-soaked wood. We sat in a circle around the embers of the fires
and made believe the cattails were cigars and put them to our
mouths and then waved them around and puffed out our chests like
gangsters in old movies. We traced circles of red-orange light with
them in the darkness.

That fall a strong, late-season storm blew in off the Atlantic. The
wind rose early one Saturday morning and carried on it the sharp,
keen scent of salt air. Seagulls flew in and circled high above the
house, wheeling and crying to each other over the rising gale. Buoy
bells out in the sound clanged furiously in a loud discordant chorus.
My brother and sister and I watched, fascinated, from the bedroom
window as the wind whipped the surface of the Sound into white
caps and pushed the high tide up over the white sandy strip of beach.
The tide slowly filled the marsh, crept up the street and then up the
steps of the front porch toward the doorsill. My mother called frantically to my father that the cellar was filled almost to its ceiling with
seawater. My father tried to reply, but he had lost his voice. Mr.
Benway called to us from outside the front door where he waited in
his boat. We cruised away from Benson Place toward higher ground
on the Old Post Road and spent the afternoon with the other neighbors at the Town Hall, waiting for the water to recede with the tide.
At the end of the day we walked back up Beach Road and over to
Benson Place. The lawns had turned brown from the seawater that
had covered them, and the heavy smell of brine hung in the air.
Along the way, neighbors were hauling furniture and soaked carpets
out into their yards but the water had stopped at the top step of our
front porch and, except for the cellar, the house was dry and clean.
The Websters, neighbors across the street, spent the next few nights
with us, and my mother took turns with Mrs. Webster, getting up in
the night to feed and change her new baby.

My Grandmother Ryan came to stay with us that first Christmas.
She slept in her old big four-poster bed that my sister and I now

shared, and we slept on two cots. Two days before Christmas, my father bought a tall Christmas tree and strung the big, colored Christmas lights on it. My mother went up into the attic and brought down the old glass ornaments that my father's mother had saved from her childhood Christmases in Germany. My Grandmother Ryan popped big bowls of popcorn, and my brother and sister and I strung the crunchy kernels on long pieces of stiff thread and wound them around the tree. We cut strips from red and green construction paper and pasted them together into long paper chains and draped the tree with those. We hung our stockings on the real fireplace and went to bed. In the middle of the night, my sister woke me to whisper that our parents were still up.

"How can Santa come if they're still in the living room? What are they doing down there?"

"Hush," said my Grandmother from her big bed. "Go to sleep or Santa will hear you!"

"But they're up!"

"Be still now. Hush!"

"I can't sleep!"

"Try."

In the darkness, I could see out of the window and up at a star-filled sky.

"Gram?"

"What?"

"What time do you think he was born?"

"Who?"

"The baby Jesus."

"He was born at midnight. Go to sleep."

My sister crawled out of bed and went over to the window.

"What are you doing? I told you to go to sleep!"

"Where is the Christmas star?"

"Wherever you can see it."

I got up and went to the window.

"There are so many! Which one is it?"

"The biggest one. Go to bed!"

Two days after Christmas, the sky turned dark gray early in the morning and the air smelled of cold iron. The milkman hurried around the house to the back porch and banged on the door for my mother. He handed her our three quarts of milk. "They'll freeze solid if you don't bring them in," he told her. "Big weather blowing in." My mother took the bottles of milk and poured off the cream from the top for my grandmother's tea. They sat together at the kitchen table and drank their tea and watched out the back window as a biting, frigid wind came up and moved through the marsh grasses. The wind whistled faintly through the bare branches of the maple trees in front. Outside, one of the shutters on the garage window began to slap against the side of the garage. My father came home early from work. He went out and fastened the shutters tightly against the garage window. The snow began to fall in the early afternoon in small, delicate flakes that whirled in the air and swept across the road and the driveways like small clouds of dry, white dust before the rising wind. Within an hour, the snow was falling so heavily that we couldn't see the house across the street. By nightfall the wind outside howled through the gables of our house and rattled the windows. I rushed out onto the back porch and felt the strength of the wind and the stinging snow on my face and the bitter cold. I stood transfixed, in my nightgown, hanging on to the porch railing as the white storm swirled around the corners of our house, past the porch and over the marsh. My mother screamed at me from the kitchen door.

"Get in here! You are too small! The wind will pick you up and carry you away with it!"

But I stood paralyzed on the porch and stared straight up into the storm and the spinning white flakes. I raised my bare arms up into the frigid wind. I stuck my tongue out and caught the snowflakes on it. My father came out, picked me up under his arm and carried me back into the kitchen.

"You should have your head examined!"

"I can't help it," I screamed. "I love it!"

"Well, love it from inside the house where it's safe."

"It's not the same! Besides, I can take care of myself!"

I looked over at my grandmother, smiling at the kitchen table.

"Here," she said, patting the chair next to her. "Have a cup of tea with me."

The snow fell for two days and nights. Only yellow flashing lights announced the big snowplows as they came through the swirling whiteness. The snow muffled all sound except the wind. It moaned and then shrieked and then quieted again. The storm ended the evening of the second day, and a frigid cold came down and settled with the night. The cold found its way into the old house. My father kept coal heaped in the furnace in the cellar, and my brother and I brought armloads of wood in from the garage. My grandmother sat next to the fireplace and kept the fire blazing. My mother kept the oven on in the kitchen until way after supper, and we went to bed with socks and sweaters over our flannel pajamas. The next morning, we could see our breath in front of our faces in the bedroom when we woke up. The sun rose in a sky of cobalt blue and shone on a scene of such dazzling whiteness that the light made my eyes ache. Three feet of snow lay glistening over the marsh and the beach beyond. The Sound reflected the deep, intense blue of the sky. The road was obliterated. I could not stay in the house. I waded out into thigh-high drifts and threw myself down on my back and flapped my arms up and down in the drifts and made snow angels. I pushed through the drifts to the marsh to see how the sparkling snow looked on the stubble of dried reeds and the long silvery bulrushes. I went home, changed my wet mittens and snowpants for dry ones. My hands turned red and chapped and then began to crack and bleed from the cold. My grandmother took one look at them one night and got out a blue jar of Vicks Mentholated Vapo-Rub. "Here," she said. "Put both hands in your lap." She smeared the cold salve all over them.

"Get me your white gloves."

"But it's winter!"

"Get them."

She pulled the white gloves over my tingling hands.

"Now get into bed. They'll be better in the morning and they won't hurt when you make your snowmen."

She pulled the heavy covers up around me, lifted the mattress and shoved the covers under it. Then she dropped the mattress with such force that my body bounced.

"I haven't said my prayers!"

"Say them in bed. Go to sleep."

The next spring my father bought bicycles for my brother and me. My brother's was red. Mine was maroon with chrome fenders. It had a wicker basket attached to the handlebar with leather straps. I was eleven that year. My brother was eight. And with our bicycles we were free. From that spring on, my brother and I were hardly ever home. We rode down to the beach at low tide and stared out at the lighthouse at the far end of Penfield Reef, several miles out in the sound. We calculated how long it would take us to walk out to the lighthouse and back before the tide returned and covered the reef. I had always wanted to make the walk, beat the tide. We made plans to try it.

I rode my bike down the Post Road to Hansen's florist on Mother's Day and bought my mother a gardenia to wear to Mass. She loved the deep green leaves and the velvet white petals. It was her favorite flower. She wore it all day and then put it in a small cut-glass bowl filled with water. The sweet, strong scent lingered in the house for days. I rode my bike after school over to the orchard and the beach, or along the Post Road, past the old white colonials and under the tall oak trees to the library in the center of Fairfield where I took out as many books as my bike basket would hold: *The Yearling, Little Women, The Adventures of Robinson Crusoe*. I brought my books to a place I had found at the southern end of the marsh, just where the rough saw grasses and tall rushes met the soft white sand dunes of the beach. It was a small, hollowed-out place in the sand, a kind of natural nest, protected from the wind and hidden from view, surrounded on all sides by the dunes. Wild roses and bayberry bushes covered the dunes. If I dug my hands too far into the fine, white sand though, thorns from the wild rose bushes would prick me by surprise. I could go there in every season but winter and lay in the soft sand, protected, and read. I loved this place. I took my dog, Pepper, and she ran along next to my bike as I pedaled down the marsh path to my place. She loved to lie curled next to me, in the warm sand, dozing for hours while I read, on and on.

My brother took his bike after school to the baseball field on Reef Road and to the end of South Benson Road where he went fishing off the jetty with his friends. He rode his bike to Cub Scout meetings and to Blinn's toy store on the Post Road. Sometimes my brother and I just rode quietly along the beach road, side by side, together. My father worked very hard to give us this wondrous place away from him.

CHAPTER EIGHT

The Unselfish Girl Is the Good Girl: Learning to Think of Others First

W e were enrolled in the fourth grade at Saint Thomas Catholic school, a square, two-story red brick building that stood in the middle of an asphalt schoolyard. The school was in back of the church and the convent, both of which faced the Boston Post Road, the main street of Fairfield. The rectory was on the far side of the church, on the left. This imposing gray wooden house, with wide verandas and an ornate, carved wooden front door, was once the home of a wealthy Fairfield merchant who donated it to the church. It was set way back from the street, surrounded by broad lawns and carefully tended gardens. The church separated the rectory from the convent.

Thirty-five children were in my fourth-grade class. The girls wore dark green uniforms with white blouses; the boys wore dark green pants with white shirts and dark green ties. The classroom was exactly the same as all the other Catholic schoolrooms I'd been in.

We sat in long rows of wooden desks with the seats attached. The rows faced the front of the classroom and the small platform on which sat Sister's desk. In back of the desk was a long blackboard. On the wall above it was a large wooden crucifix with a white plaster body of Christ attached to it. Drops of red paint were dabbed on the figure's chest and hands and feet.

On either side of the blackboard was a door that led into the cloakroom. This was a long, narrow closet behind the blackboard with a row of hooks for our coats and a long, low shelf underneath the hooks for our lunch boxes. At Saint Thomas, I was the "new" girl until I graduated.

In fourth grade, the nun Sister Melita wore the long black habit of the Sisters of Mercy, an Irish order of nuns known for their teaching skills and their work with the poor and downtrodden. The black habit had long sleeves and skirt and an oversized, starched white bib that covered her chest like a breastplate, protecting . . . what? Around her waist she wore a black leather belt and an oversized set of brown, wooden rosary beads that clacked together when she walked. A starched white wimple and a long black veil framed her face. Everyone knew she and the other sisters shaved their heads. The lessons were the same as all the other Catholic schools I'd attended. The day always began with prayers. The Our Father. The Hail Mary. The Apostle's Creed. The Prayer to Saint Michael the Archangel . . . "Defend us in battle against the malice and snares of the devil . . ." and then the recitations from the Baltimore catechism. Why did God make us? What is a sin?

In the fifth grade, our teacher Sister Placide was aged and kindly. She taught us decimal points and fractions and the essential points of a well-constructed sentence. She diagrammed the sentences on the blackboard and, with a long wooden pointer, showed us the position of the nouns and verbs and adverbs. Then she turned to face us and leaned back against the blackboard and explained the difference between subjects and predicates, transitive and intransitive verbs. Then she turned back to the board and began to draw more diagrams to illustrate what she had said. The white chalk lines and words she had drawn on the board appeared again, in reverse, on the back of her long black habit.

In the sixth grade, Sister Marie Pauline was our teacher. She was a stunning young woman, tall and graceful. She had deep, violet eyes and long, black lashes. Her black eyebrows swept up toward her temples like the wings of a bird. Her skin looked soft, white, silky, and in the winter, in the schoolyard, her cheeks blazed red with the cold. She wore black woolen mittens to cover her little hands. Monsignor Casey, the pastor, was a short, wiry, little man with ruddy cheeks and white hair. He began to appear in the schoolyard in his black cassock and crimson sash whenever we were at recess. Soon he was there not only at every recess, but at every lunch hour. He stood very close to Sister Marie Pauline and took her hands in his to warm them. In March, after the Easter vacation, Sister Marie Pauline was gone, and Monsignor Casey never came to the schoolyard again.

Sermons on death and denial hurried diligently after the glorious seasons of the year. With the scent of fresh, unfrozen earth and the first hint of spring came the penitential season of Lent. There were new pussy willows in the marsh and tiny green buds on the forsythia bushes, but on Ash Wednesday we marched across the schoolyard to the church where Monsignor Casey dabbed our foreheads with ashes and told each of us in Latin, "Remember that you are dust and into dust you shall return."

We prayed:

Grant us, O Lord, to begin the duties of our Christian warfare with holy fasts;
That as we do battle with the spirits of evil,
We may be protected by the help of self denial.

Good Catholics gave up that thing that was most dear for Lent. I gave up my bike. But only my bike. I walked through the marsh to the beach. I walked over to the apple trees. I walked down to the library to return my books and take more out.

At Easter time, while the air all around us was suffused with the dizzying perfume of hyacinths and lilacs, we were reminded that when we died we would be able to join Christ in heaven because he had died for us and had risen from the dead.

In summer, the priest wore vestments of green, the symbol of hope and renewal. All through the warm, carefree, soft summer season, we celebrated the feast days of virgins and martyrs, those who had died horrible deaths for their faith. My classmates and I always loved the feast day on July 17 of Saint Alexius, who was not a martyr. Our daily missals told us that he was the son of a noble Roman family who renounced all his worldly goods, and on his wedding night made a pilgrimage, alone, to Syria where he stayed, by himself, for seventeen years. When he finally returned, he lived under the stairs of his father's palace, hidden away from his father and his own wife. When he died of natural causes under the stairs in 417 A.D., papers were found on his body, which identified him. "He was immediately honored as a saint," said our missal. And probably a virgin.

For Catholics, the season of Advent occurs in the month before Christmas. The church tempers the joyful anticipation of the birth of Christ with the reminders of the fires of hell and the remembrance that we are all sinners. Christ the Redeemer was born to save us all from damnation. We prayed to be purified before his birth. At mass we prayed:

We entreat your mercy, O Lord, that having cleansed us from our vices, You may prepare us for the coming festivities. Filled with the food of this spiritual nourishment . . . You would teach us to despise earthly things and to love those of heaven.

For the Catholic child Advent was a time to pay special attention
to confession. To prepare for the coming of Christ, we had to cleanse
our souls through the Sacrament of Penance. I had always been
afraid of confession. In school, we were constantly reminded that to
omit a sin from your confession put your soul in mortal danger. The
nuns told us that if we left church after such a deliberate omission
and were struck by a car and killed, we would go straight to hell.
Since the teaching of the church during Advent was "to despise
earthly things and to love those of heaven," I thought it must be sin-
ful to look forward to receiving gifts for Christmas. Presents were
"earthly" things, weren't they? But it was difficult to spend Saturday
afternoon shopping with my mother for Christmas presents for my
grandmother and my aunts without wondering what my parents
might have bought for my brother and sister and me. It was really difficult because we always stopped at the church for Saturday afternoon confession before we went home. Should I tell the priest my
thoughts about Christmas presents? I was absolutely terrified of leaving anything out. I knew you had to tell the priest everything that
might be a sin. My mother tried to clear up my confusion. "Just think
about what you'll be giving to others rather than what you'll be getting for yourself."

"But do I tell the priest that I don't despise earthly things? Do I tell
him I am selfish?"

"If you think about yourself first, yes. You are selfish."

So I would wait, nervously, on the side aisle of the darkening
church, a young girl in a blue woolen cap, long coat and mittens. I
trembled, not from the cold, but in fear of making a bad confession.
My nervousness grew more extreme as my turn came to enter the
dark, little box. The lines for confession were always long, and the
old church grew dim, then dark and colder. As I waited, I searched
my mind desperately for every other sin I might have committed during the last week. I tried to uncover every nuance of my behavior. I

dreaded kneeling down in the dark, stifling box and telling some man I didn't even know my innermost thoughts. But you had to tell the priest all your sins, even if you weren't sure they were sins.

"Bless me Father for I have sinned. I have been selfish. I have thought of what I would get for Christmas before I thought of the gifts I would give."

"The good Catholic girl is an unselfish girl. Her first thought should be for others. Though we will not celebrate the feast of Christ's birth for two more weeks, you should remember that he died for us. He spent his life thinking of others first. Go now, and say your penance."

At six o'clock, when confessions were finally over, we drove home through the cold dusk of the early winter night. I set the table and helped my mother make a hurried dinner. After the dishes were done, my mother asked me to help her wrap the Christmas presents she'd bought for my grandmother and my aunts, but I was afraid the wrappings and ribbon and tissue paper would remind me again of my selfishness so I asked her to excuse me. I tried to watch "Your Show of Shows" on the new television set in the living room, but I couldn't keep myself awake. I climbed the stairs, struggled out of my clothes into pajamas, made an extra act of contrition, put all thoughts about Christmas presents out of my head and fell sound asleep.

Sister Bernard Marie, tall, thin and excitable, was my seventh-grade teacher. She had a narrow face imprisoned in her white wimple, small, distrustful eyes and red, pockmarked skin. She lost her temper, more and more, as the school year wore on. She avoided the tall boys who sat in the back of the classroom. She always called instead on the shorter, smaller boys who sat in front.

I sat in the middle row, two seats from the front. The boy who sat in back of me, Charlie Borosky, began to tap me on the shoulder when Sister's back was turned. "I like your eyes," he said when I turned around. He began to pass me notes that read, "Dear Cat's

Eyes, Can I ride my bike over to your house?" I would turn around to tell him "Ssssh," and the nun would scold me for talking. One day she sent a note home to my parents. "Susan is distracted during class by the boy who sits in back of her. When I ask her to stop talking to him and pay attention she stares at me in a very bold manner." This was the first reprimand, either written or spoken that I'd ever received in school, and strangely, I didn't care. I lost myself in the subjects I was learning, and if the school day was unpleasant, I knew I'd be out on the beach or on my bicycle after three o'clock anyway. I did tell my mother my side of the story, and she believed me, but she said, "Just don't look at her when she scolds you."

"But I'm not talking! It's Charlie!" I said.

"You know that and I know that," she said. "But there isn't much you can do about it. You're the one who aggravates her."

I went to school the next day and told Charlie to stop passing notes to me. I resolved never to look at Sister Bernard Marie in the face again. But I noticed that I wasn't the only one of the girls in my class who was having a hard time of it with the nun. Agatha Martinez was a beautiful, dark-haired Spanish girl who was new in the class that year. She was even taller than Sister Bernard Marie and when she stood up in class to answer a question, she looked down at the nun. She made Sister nervous. One afternoon, Agatha gave the correct answer to a geography question, and Sister told her she was wrong. The rest of us were shocked. Someone tittered in the back of the room. The nun whirled around to see who made the sound. "Who laughed?" she said. No one answered. Now she screamed, "Who laughed?"

"No one is laughing, Sister," said Agatha, looking down at her.

"What?" screamed the nun. "What? Who gave you permission to speak to me?"

"I don't need permission to speak to you, Sister," said Agatha, coolly.

The nun drew back her fist and hit the girl, hard, on the side of her face. Agatha staggered backward but grabbed the corner of her desk for support. She stood for a moment and then pushed the nun aside. She walked slowly toward the front of the classroom and the door to the cloakroom. The nun went after her. She shoved Agatha into the cloakroom and slammed the door. For a moment we heard nothing, but then the sound of a powerful slap rang out followed by a thudding noise on the wall in back of the blackboard. The geography map that had been drawn down to cover the blackboard crashed to the floor. Suddenly the door to the cloakroom swung open, and Agatha stormed out with her coat. She shouted back into the cloakroom over her shoulder.

"That's the last time you hit me, you pimply faced moron!"

She put on the coat and walked out of the classroom. There was no sound at all from the cloakroom.

Moments later, Sister Bernard Marie emerged and stood, leaning against the doorframe. A large, red blotch covered one side of her face. She was crying. She ran out of the room, her long, black veil streaming after her, leaving us stunned and horrified. What could possibly come next? And what would happen to Agatha's soul? She had struck a nun—a bride of Christ!

A half hour went by. Suddenly Agatha reappeared in the doorway with her mother. One of the tall boys in the back of the room stood up and cheered. "Yay, Agatha!"

"Get every last book out of your desk," said Agatha's mother. "You will not stay in this place."

Sister Bernard Marie never returned to our classroom. We never learned what happened to her. Monsignor Casey stayed with us that afternoon until the bell rang and we were dismissed. The next day we had a lay teacher, a small, plump woman named Mrs. Cronin, who took our class for the next few weeks until school recessed for the summer.

When the school year resumed the next fall for eighth grade, I began to study early in the year for the entrance exam to Lauralton Hall, a Catholic convent school for girls in the nearby town of Milford, a short train ride away from Fairfield. My parents had decided that I would attend this all-girl's school, even though the tuition was expensive. The entrance test was rigorous, and I was worried about the math section of it because I had no ease or proficiency in algebra, which we were learning.

One autumn morning as I got off the school bus, three of the bigger girls in my class met me at the entrance to the schoolyard. They were at the center of a clique of girls whose breasts had begun to "develop," and they usually stood together in a group, talking about boys and pointing at the rest of us smaller girls who were still jumping rope or playing hopscotch in the schoolyard. I was preoccupied with an algebra problem that I hadn't been able to solve the night before, and I worried that the problem might appear on a surprise quiz. I had good grades, and I couldn't afford to let one drop.

"Susan!" called one of the girls. "Do you know the facts of life?"

"No," I said. "Did we have to know those for homework?"

All three girls whooped and screamed with laughter. At lunch time I still couldn't figure out why they were laughing. I asked one of my friends.

"What are the facts of life?"

She stared at me.

"You don't know?"

"No," I said.

"Susan," she leaned close to my ear. "They're sex."

"Oh!" I said. "Why do they call sex that?"

"Sssh!" hissed my friend. She looked quickly around the lunchroom. "What?!"

"Don't ever say 'sex' out loud! What will people think?"

"Of what?" I said.

"Of you!"

"I don't care."

"I don't care never has a home."

I remembered my Grandmother's reply to that. "I don't care doesn't need one."

I didn't care. I didn't care what anyone thought. I had been reading historical romances all summer. I'd spent long summer days at the beach losing myself in the stories of love affairs of kings and queens and mistresses. It seemed to me the big girls in my class were just discovering something that had been going on for a very long time.

At dinner that night, I told my mother what the girls had said.

"Is that what they're talking about in the schoolyard?" asked my father.

"I don't know what they talk about," I said. "I'm just telling you what they asked me. It's too bad they haven't read Catherine."

"Oh?" said my father. "And what's that about?"

"John of Gaunt." Something told me not to mention that the book was about Catherine Swynford, his mistress.

"Who is John of Gaunt?"

"Was," I said. "He was the Duke of Lancaster in England and his son was Henry IV. One of his descendants founded the Tudor dynasty."

"The Tudors?"

I laughed.

"Dad! You know! Henry the VIII was a Tudor!"

"Why don't you read your algebra book instead of these stories of make-believe?"

I looked at him. I thought he was joking.

"Is that the same bold look you give to the nun in school?" he said.

"Dad! They aren't make-believe stories!"

"Shut up! That nun would probably like to give you a good smack!"

"She's just telling you what she's reading," said my mother.

"Why doesn't she tell me who'll be paying the money for her damned tuition?"

"Dad!" I said. "I don't have to go to Lauralton Hall! I'll get good grades wherever I go."

"What makes you think you're so damned smart?"

"I am smart," I said.

"Don't you dare talk back to me," he shouted. "Who do you think you are? You're a damned brat, that's who you are. And you don't care who thinks so!"

"No, I don't care," I said. "Because I know I'm not a brat."

"You are a damned ungrateful brat!" he screamed. He was livid. He banged his fists on the table so that the plates jumped. "Get out! Get out of my sight!"

I was shocked. I got up from the table, went out to the garage, got on my bike and rode down to the beach. I sat on the beach and stared out over the Sound until it began to get dark and the light far out at the end of Penfield Reef began to beam on and off across the water. I knew I wasn't a brat. But what did he mean by ungrateful? Was I being selfish? I knew he and my mother wanted to buy their own house. I'd overheard them talking about it. I sensed he was nervous about that. I didn't have to go to Lauralton Hall. I didn't want to go there anyway. I wanted to go to the public high school. I was only going because he and my mother wanted me to. He didn't have to pay my tuition, especially when he was worried about affording the new house. I decided that I would tell him he didn't have to send me there. I felt guilty, somehow. I couldn't understand why. What was I costing him? Was it too much?

I pedaled home. He was sitting in the living room.

"I'm sorry, Dad," I said. "I don't have to go to that school. I know you're worried about the new house."

"You're not that smart that you know what I'm thinking. Try not to be so selfish. Good night."

That fall, when I was in the eighth grade, Charlie Borosky did ride his bike over to my house, and so did several other boys. He lounged around in the front yard and I assumed he'd come over to see my brother, who was on the same baseball team with him. But he and the other boys stayed in the front yard when my brother rode off on his bike. They talked among themselves and Charley kept looking sideways over at me as I sat on the front porch with my friend Janie who lived next door. One Friday afternoon he asked me to meet him at the Community Theatre the next afternoon.

"All the kids go to the movies on Saturdays," he said.

"I don't," I said.

"We could sit together," he said.

"No thank you," I said. "I sat in front of you in school last year. That nun sent a note home to my parents about me because of you."

"Old red-face sent a note home? Because of me?" He was shocked.

"Yes, and I don't want any more notes from anybody. I told you that last year, too. Besides, I go sailing on Saturdays."

He looked disappointed, and he blushed. I thought I'd hurt his feelings.

"I'm sorry, Charlie," I said. "It isn't you. I just would rather go sailing." I didn't realize then that Charlie was the first boy who had a sexual interest in me. I didn't know why he wanted to be near me.

Early Saturday mornings I pedaled my bike over to Ash Creek where one of the lifeguards I knew from the beach was teaching me to sail. We'd take his old wooden boat out into the open water of the Sound, and then I'd climb aft and take the rudder in one hand and the rope of the frayed canvas sail in the other. He taught me how to come about into the wind so that the sail luffed and then filled, and we were off, running before the wind, skimming along the surface of the open Sound. The only sounds were of the water as it rushed along the sides of the little boat and the cries of the gulls as they wheeled in circles high overhead.

He taught me how to sail the little boat into the wind on an oblique, zigzag path called tacking. First we tacked to starboard, then to port, until we reached a destination, usually one of the buoy bells that were anchored out, parallel to shore. "Now don't worry about what might happen," he told me. "Don't be afraid of the unexpected. Be prepared for it. If you're in control, you can handle it. It takes longer to sail against the wind because all the time you're beating ahead, the wind and the currents are beating you back. Trim your sail and take the rudder with a firm hand. Don't give up. If you let out too much sail, the wind will blow you over. You have to keep your balance otherwise you'll capsize and go down."

Late that winter, on a gray morning in February, the air turned humid and chilly and a freezing rain began to fall. We were let out of school at noon and my father came home early from work. The house was cold and damp. He went down to the cellar and shoveled more coal into the furnace, then he got wood in and started a fire in the fireplace, but the house seemed to resist all his efforts. The chill was too deep.

By late afternoon, a thick coating of ice lay over the marsh grasses and flattened them. Ice encased the branches of the maple trees, and they bent, almost to the ground, under the weight of it. Of course I had to go out. But I couldn't go further than the front step. The limbs of the maples swayed and made a light tinkling sound like glass chimes in the chill, soft wind. Pieces of the ice fell and skittered across the ice cover of the street. Suddenly, I heard a loud crack in one of the maple trees in the front of the house. A huge limb snapped and tore away from the tree and fell heavily to the street, leaving a raw white gash on the brown trunk. I sat by myself on the front step and watched other limbs of the maples crack and fall until the broken, brown branches, still in their icy coverings, were lying in tangled heaps all over the icy crust on the street, and all the beautiful maples were splintered, scarred, raw. I heard all around me, from far across the marsh, the sound of other trees groaning and breaking, then smashing on the ground.

I passed the entrance exam to Lauralton Hall the next spring and our eighth-grade class prepared to graduate. In May, we had the usual Crowning of the Blessed Virgin Mother ceremony, and we got our white graduation dresses early so we could wear them in the May Procession. Under the white dresses we wore slips and garter belts and stockings that had seams running up the backs. My mother had to help me with the intricacies of adjusting the hooks on the garter belts and then fastening the tops of the stockings to the hooks. These new clothes felt awkward and scratchy, but somehow grown-up. I had grown taller but no fuller, and while all my friends wore bras under their white dresses, I didn't. My grandmother made me camisoles instead.

"Oh!" I said to her one day. "I wish I had big breasts!"

"Wish in one hand and spit in the other," she said. "See what you get first."

"If you're worried," said my mother, "maybe you could wear falsies."

"What are falsies?"

"Gay Deceivers," said my grandmother. "You put them in your camisole so they look like you have breasts."

"What?" I screamed. "That's ridiculous!"

During that spring of 1953, my mother and father bought a small lot on a street across the marsh from us, just off Beach Road. The lot was close to the beach, just a short walk away. They planned to build a long, low ranch-style house on it, the first house they had ever owned. I was sad to think of leaving Benson Place, but we would just be living on the far side of the marsh. That and the beach were always the same peaceful places for me. Every night after dinner, my parents would drive over to see the progress on the new house. My father was preoccupied and nervous about moving. He worried, even more than usual, about money.

On Saturday afternoons during that spring of 1953, I started to walk down to the Center of Fairfield to meet my friends at the Community Theatre to watch the double features. We watched Audrey Hepburn and Gregory Peck in *Roman Holiday* and James Mason and Ava Gardner in *Pandora and the Flying Dutchman*. Afterwards we walked to Clampett's drugstore on the Post Road and sipped cherry cokes. We wore short-sleeved blouses and full skirts with wide belts and crinoline petticoats underneath to make the skirts look even fuller. We wore little black ballerina slippers called Capezios. We had just started to listen to music on the jukebox, "Only You" by The Platters, and "Rock Around the Clock" by Bill Haley and his Comets. We sang along with Gene Vincent and his Blue Cats . . .

Be Bop a Lula, she's my baby,
Be Bop a Lula, don't mean maybe . . .

Several of my friends had started to wear lipstick. The Saturday before graduation, my mother and I went into Clampett's drugstore where she bought me a tube of Coty Girl pale pink lipstick. We went home and upstairs to look in the bathroom mirror and put it on. My mother stood behind me in the mirror as I carefully traced the lipstick onto my lips. She showed me in the mirror how to press my lips together to make sure the lipstick covered evenly. I looked in the mirror at myself. The color on my mouth made everything about my reflection more vivid. My lips looked full and bright, and my eyes were very pale blue in the mirror. They were exactly the color of my grandmother's eyes. The lipstick made my hair and my eyelashes look even darker, and I noticed that my eyebrows slanted upwards. I suddenly understood why Charlie Borosky had called me "cat's eyes."

"What's the matter?" my mother said.

"I don't know," I said.

"Of course you do," she said. "You look absolutely beautiful! Just show Dad!"

She called to my father who was in their bedroom.

"Look how beautiful Susan looks with her lipstick on!"

I went out into the hall to show my father. He came out of his room, and I smiled at him. He slapped me across my mouth with such force that I slammed against the opposite wall of the hall and fell, halfway back into the bathroom. My mother screamed. My brother ran out of his bedroom and rushed headlong at my father and knocked him to the floor. He sat on my father. My mother, still screaming, pulled my brother away from my father. My father sat up on the hall floor and looked around himself, dazed. I got up and fled down the stairs, sobbing. My brother screamed after me.

"Susan! Susan! Go!"

I ran, sobbing, out of the house and through the gate at the end of the street. I ran down the wide, white sandy path and cut into the marsh. I hid myself among the tall grasses and made my way through them to my secret place. I threw myself down in the soft sand and crawled in among the wild roses and bayberry bushes to cover myself. The wild rose bushes scratched and tore at my bare legs and arms. I felt the greasy, pink lipstick smeared across my mouth and cheek. I sobbed. "Why? What have I done? What is wrong with me?" But the marsh held no answers.

&&&&&

How could I have known that on that long-ago day I was beginning to lose myself?

CHAPTER NINE

Bernie Siegel: Day Four

I awoke on the day after the hemorrhage feeling more rested and calm than I had been in months, and although my chest was sore, I couldn't feel that anything was missing. Pat was coming with Annie that morning, a Saturday. He would drive the fifty miles from Fairfield to Wallingford, pick her up and bring her to see me in New Haven, bring her back to Choate, and on his way back to Fairfield stop in and see me again.

As I read more of the Simontons' book I noticed that they'd mentioned another book that they called one of the finest studies on the relationship between emotional states and cancer. This was *A Psychological Study of Cancer*, written by a Dr. Elida Evans and published in 1926. A student of the Swiss psychiatrist Carl Jung, Dr. Evans had made a detailed study of the emotional states of 100 cancer patients before the onset of their disease. I wanted to read the book, but it was out of print. However, it had been published by

Dodd, Mead and Company in New York, which was also Pat's publisher. He asked one of his editors there to track it down, and he'd gone into New York to get it for me.

I could hear Annie's laughter all the way down the hall. I smiled at the sound of it. She burst into my room, draped her arms carefully around me and kissed me. "Mom!" she said, "everyone wants to know when you're coming home! No one can get away with anything while you're gone!"

She sat on the edge of my bed, long legs dangling, and within minutes was regaling me and Pat and a small crowd of captivated nurses, who had somehow gathered into the room, with stories of some of her classmates at school. Annie still wasn't aware of the delightful effect of her irrepressible laughter and easy charm. Before dawn that very morning, she told us, one of the freshman girls was caught shinnying down from the second floor of the dormitory. She'd climbed down, almost past a teacher's open bedroom window, when she realized she hadn't tied enough sheets together and her "rope" was too short. The teacher woke and saw a pair of naked legs thrashing in front of the window. The girl swayed slowly, back and forth ("at the end of her rope!" roared Annie) while the teacher went out and waited for her to drop to the ground.

Now Annie began on her favorite story, "Beatrice and the Bong." This was about me and my first week as a "dorm mother" in the freshman girls' dormitory. One of my duties was to check the girls' rooms at ten each night to make sure everyone was in bed with lights out. When I went in to Beatrice's room, the lights were out, and she and her roommate were in their beds. I smelled an exotic, smoky fragrance in the room, which I thought was incense. As I turned to leave I tripped over something on the floor. I turned the light on and saw what looked like a round vase lying on the floor. Beatrice lay absolutely still in her bed, her eyes fixed on me. The other girl pulled her covers up over her head. "Beatrice," I said, "what is this lovely vase doing on the floor?" Now Beatrice eyed me suspiciously.

"I don't know," she said. "Maybe it just rolled there?"

"Well," I said, "try to take better care of your things. Good night, girls."

A few days later, when I told Annie the story, she said, "I know, Mom. Beatrice told everyone. She keeps wondering when you're going to turn her in."

"Why would I turn her in?"

"You tripped over her bong, Mom."

"Her bong? What is a bong?"

Annie gave out a long sigh and regarded me with sympathy.

"It's for smoking grass, Mom." Then she added hopefully, "You know . . . marijuana?"

"Oh, my God," I said.

By now the nurses were doubled over with laughter.

"You're a dorm mother?" asked Rita. "How long will that job last?"

"It isn't a problem!" shrieked Annie. "Everyone else loves my mother! Beatrice is the only one who's scared of her!"

Annie told me the latest family news. Her father would be coming to see me with Andrew tomorrow. Someone from the hospital had tried to call my former husband yesterday when I had hemorrhaged. Andrew had answered the phone for Harry, who was out. The person told him that his mother was critically ill and that the hospital needed to notify a close family member. Andrew was horrified. Now he insisted on coming to see me with his father. Dana had already called me twice from California to make sure I was fine. I still had not heard anything from Peggy. I couldn't understand why.

Thanksgiving vacation started the next week, and I wanted to be home at Choate by then. Annie would spend Thanksgiving with me. Dana would be with friends in California. Andrew was spending Thanksgiving with his father. I still didn't know Peggy's plans. I'd been divorced for two years now, but the holidays were still grueling affairs and I dreaded them. These were the days when families were supposed to be together. I looked at Annie draped across the foot of my bed, and my heart went out to her. I couldn't help the tears stinging in my eyes. What had I done? How could I have broken up my family?

Annie noticed instantly.

"Mom!" she cried out. "What's wrong?"

"Nothing!" I lied. "I'm just so sorry that I upset everyone. I'm fine now. I really am."

Pat had been taking all this in.

"You didn't upset everyone, Susan," he said quietly. "You couldn't help a hemorrhage. It's not your fault that you got sick."

"I know," I said. But I couldn't keep myself from thinking that it was.

As Annie and Pat were leaving, she leaned over to kiss me good-bye. I could see that she was perspiring. I suddenly realized how hard she'd worked to entertain everyone. She whispered anxiously to me.

"Mom, are you going to be okay?"

"Absolutely," I said.

"Okay," she said. "But I'm going to call you every day." I understood how she'd tried to please. She'd delighted everyone else, but her first question, that which was most important to her, was the one she saved for last. "Mom, are you going to be okay?" Why did she wait to whisper that question? Why were other people more important than her own needs? Had she lost her sense of self? Had she learned that lesson from me? Afraid of displeasing, afraid to think of myself first? And the one time that I had thought of myself I had caused anguish and loss for everyone I loved. I thought of the old lesson: "The good girl is the unselfish girl." But I had been selfish.

Lost in my thoughts, I was startled to see Dr. McCullough and another doctor standing next to my bed. He was a short, trim man with the compact bearing of a military officer. He seemed full of a tightly contained energy, like a small, shiny bullet.

"Susan," said Dr. McCullough, "here's someone you'll enjoy meeting. This is Dr. Siegel."

"Bernie," said the little man. "Call me Bernie."

He smiled at me, a broad, happy grin, and reached out to shake my hand. He wore a Mickey Mouse watch.

"Hi, Dr. Siegel," I said. I couldn't bring myself to call a doctor by his first name. "Thank you for the book by the Simontons."

"You're welcome," he said. "Did you read it?"

"Yes," I said. "I read the whole thing."

He looked absolutely delighted.

"I'll leave you two," said Dr. McCullough. "See you tomorrow."

"So, how are you?" asked Bernie.

"Fine," I said. "Well, no. Not really."

"What's going on?"

"I was just thinking about what the Simontons wrote about learning to ask for things for yourself. My daughter was just here to visit, and I can see that she puts other people's needs before her own. I'm afraid she learned that from me."

"Is that what you believe?"

"I always thought it was selfish to think of myself first," I said.

He didn't respond. Then he said, suddenly, "Do you wear your seat belt in the car?"

"What?"

"I want to know if you wear your seat belt in the car."

What kind of question is this? I thought. *And from a doctor?* "No," I said. "I have to admit I don't."

"Well, you should. Because when you put it on you're saying three things to yourself. One, you love yourself enough to protect yourself. Two, you want to be in control of yourself, even if someone else should hit your car. Three, you love yourself enough to concentrate on the future! It's okay to love yourself, you know."

"I'm trying to unlearn some of the things I believed all my life," I said. "It's difficult."

"True," he said. "And important. I think you'll do fine. Are you doing your visualizations?"

"Yes. I've got a whole army set up in my immune system."

He laughed. "Good! Because a good vivid mental picture can cause your body to change for the better. The body thinks the wonderful thing you're imagining is the real thing! And keep reading!" He patted my foot for emphasis and went out.

Rita came in to take my blood pressure. "I see you met Dr. Siegel," she said, smiling. "He's quite a character. You lucked out with both those guys."

"Why do you say that?" I said.

"He and Dr. McCullough are just a few of the doctors around here who don't think M.D. after their names means medical deity. Bernie believes patients have more power than they think. He really believes that sometimes patients can heal themselves."

"Do you think that?" I said.

She paused. "I probably shouldn't say this," she said, "but a lot of the doctors I meet don't bother much with the patient. They're only interested in the illness. That makes patients scared, like they're all alone and helpless. Bernie's patients feel like they have some kind of control. Dr. McCullough's patients are usually calmer than others. He makes them feel special."

"That's true," I said. I remembered him standing outside the operating room, waiting for me. "I feel that way."

All doctors should treat their patients with the same care, I thought. Most doctors studied bodies as specimens, as "cases," as if the body did not belong to the patient. They rarely considered the whole person, much less any emotional turmoil that person may have been suffering. I remembered the first doctor I'd seen in New York. He had no interest in me. He had made a name for himself fighting the illness.

"Why does Dr. Siegel like people to call him Bernie?" I asked.

"So they know he's human like they are."

I remembered what he'd said: "The event is not in charge, you are. That's when you have power." His philosophy of self-control fit the way he looked. He obviously took good care of himself. I remembered his compact little frame. I guessed that he watched his weight, and I was sure he went to a gym and worked out. *He's in charge of himself*, I thought. He'd said, "Keep concentrating on the very best. And keep reading!" As he suggested, I picked up the book Pat had brought me and began to read.

∽∂∾∂∾∂

Elida Evans began her psychological research with cancer patients at Carl Jung's School of Analytic Psychology, in Zurich, Switzerland, in 1921. Jung, her mentor, had just published a book called *Psychological Types* in which he introduced the concept of certain types of people, the introvert and the extravert. The extravert is the person whose psychological well-being is totally dependent on external things or people. This type of person wears a "persona" (from the Latin word meaning mask, or role) in order to please people and to adapt or "fit in" to the requirements of his or her environment.

The introvert is the opposite: this person doesn't need a mask. Introverts don't depend on others' approval. They don't care what other people think. They are self-reliant, strong and secure within themselves.

Evans was curious to see if there was a certain psychological trait among her cancer patients. "They have not been the helpless ones in the beginning," she wrote. "They have started out with full force and it has not been grief alone which stopped them. They have had a peculiar sorrow and a special temperament with which to meet it."

She took what she called "mental, emotional histories" of each over a five-year period. Her research revealed not only that all the cancer patients had similar histories, but that all were extraverts, people whose health, happiness and security depended on people or objects outside themselves. "The extravert draws his life sustaining energy from the object to whom he is attached, whether a human being, a professional or a business interest," she observed, "and when separated from the object he is lost." Like the Simontons, Evans theorized that it is this "loss" that weakens the body and spirit, making it susceptible to the disease. I remembered that the Simontons, too, had theorized that cancer was somehow associated with how particular people view loss.

But, wrote Evans, "I have never found a case of carcinoma among the introverted type." Strong "individuals" are independent people who don't live for others; they are entirely secure within themselves. For Jung and Evans, then, the introvert was the stronger person. These are people who see loss as part of the ebb and flow of a normal life.

I'd never really understood the meaning of the word "introvert." I'd always thought that to be an introvert meant you were a shy, "withdrawn" fragile person, almost a negative trait. Now I was realizing that introverts are the strong individuals who, according to Evans, find themselves in opposition to the "collective authority," or as my mother would have said, "what everybody thinks." I knew this was true. When I was a young girl in school, to be an "individual" meant that you were odd, "different" from everyone else. You didn't fit in. Other girls put their fingers over their mouths and whispered about you to one another. You weren't part of "the collective authority," the clique or the crowd.

I remembered the extraverted girls, the ones with "personality." They were "outgoing," the "life of the party." They were exciting figures, and they always had groups around them. They were always part of the clique, the "collective authority," and looking back, they seemed to need those cliques. But in those days, being an outsider didn't frighten me. When I was a young schoolgirl I never cared what others thought.

In later years, I lost my individuality and my inner-strength. Now I was realizing that I fit the definition of extravert. I'd learned to put on a mask, to assume a role—dutiful daughter, wife and mother—because I was frightened of displeasing the people who were so important to me. Like anyone who lives to please, I believed that others' wishes were more important than mine and I was helpless without approval. I'd become afraid of standing on my own, of being "different," of not "fitting in."

But there was that time in my childhood when I was strong, when I was an individual—an introvert—for a time. I had learned, on my own, how to live securely within myself, to think for myself. I'd been strong enough to say, "I don't care. . . . I am in control." How could I get back to the child I once was? How had I lost my self-strength? I had to know, for now I had to make sure that I understood for Annie's sake as well.

CHAPTER TEN

Losing Myself

At Lauralton Hall, when I was fourteen, Annie's age, the focus of sin had shifted ever so slightly from selfishness and landed squarely on top of sex. Lauralton, set in an old stone mansion and the lovely gardens of the estate that surrounded it, had once been the home of a wealthy spinster. She died and left the house and grounds to the Sisters of Mercy, who now ran it as a school. This was the same order of nuns that had been my teachers in grammar school. These women were even more intense and watchful than the women who had disciplined us as children. They were responsible for protecting the virtue of 200 teenage girls, and our parents paid sizable tuitions for that protection. The nuns took very good care of us for that money. They controlled us absolutely. They were merciless.

We wore navy-blue serge jumpers with white blouses underneath, brown oxfords and white socks. There were no deviations from the uniform. Joan Reynolds, one of the girls with "flair" came to school one day wearing brown and white saddle shoes and was immediately sent home to change them. We were forbidden to look different. We had to appear "uniform"—the same.

The navy-blue jumpers had a sash that you could tie in back so that you could show off your waist, but we were not allowed to tie the sashes too tightly because then the uniform would show our breasts, which could be "occasions of sin." At fifteen, I was tall and thin, but I had finally developed breasts. Like a knowledge I didn't want, I had them. They were full, round and painful. They were embarrassing. People stared at them. They were probably occasions of sin.

The nuns lectured us constantly on occasions of sin. The most perilous of these was, of course, sex. Sex was everywhere because it was not allowed anywhere. We read *MacBeth*, but not *Romeo and Juliet*. We read Emily Dickenson but not Walt Whitman. In Latin class, we translated Caesar's *Gallic Wars*, but not the love poetry of Catallus:

Kiss me now a thousand times and then a hundred more
And then a hundred and a thousand more again,
'Til with so many hundred thousand kisses
You and I shall both lose count, nor any can for envy of so much kissing,
Put his finger on the number of sweet kisses,
You of me, and I of you, darling, have had.

So, while Julius Caesar was busy dividing Gaul into three parts, Catallus was bestowing hundreds of thousands of kisses upon his beloved. But we didn't read that. Sex probably meant freedom. We never read of freedom.

Sex. Sex. Sex. They warned us of nothing else. What else was there? Sex! All the nuns talked about was the punishment for it and the necessity of avoiding it. And the more they talked about it, the more interesting it became. The very idea of it was overpowering, inescapable in the school. How could one think of anything but sex? Well, you could become a nun.

Once a week each of us met with Sister Denise, the guidance counselor.

"Susan, have you ever considered entering the convent?" This was always her first question.

"No, Sister." This was always what I answered.

"Why not?"

"I don't want to become a nun."

"But God may be calling you."

"Yes, Sister, but I don't want to go."

Three times a year we were required to attend retreat. Classes were suspended for three days, and we spent those days in the chapel in quiet meditation, interrupted only by sermons on the "impurities" of sex. The sermons during retreat were devoted to descriptions of hell and its unspeakable, fiery torments. Mother Superior chose the priest who would conduct the retreat and give these frightening sermons. The most compelling speaker got the job. Since he would spend three days at the convent, waited on by a bevy of excited nuns and two hundred teen-aged girls, the competition was fierce among priests, and the sermons got more terrifying—and as we matured, more sexually explicit. There he would stand, Father Anselm, the Dominican, all austerity in his white robe, his eyes hidden by the folds of his black cowl, preaching in front of a rapt audience of pubescent girls.

The nuns conducted question-and-answer sessions on the intricacies of the Sixth Commandment. Father Anselm sat in and listened.

"Thou shalt not commit adultery." This commandment would seem to apply only to those who were married, but no. The Sixth Commandment applied to anyone over the age of reason. For an order of nuns assigned to run a school for Catholic girls, the Sixth Commandment was a weapon of sexual control.

Question: "What if I were kissing a boy and I allowed him to touch my breasts and we were killed on our way home from our date?"

Answer: "Not only would you go straight to hell, but you would be responsible for the loss of your boyfriend's soul as well because you did not stop him from committing a sin. A good confession would have cleansed your souls and allowed you both into heaven, but of course you did not have the opportunity for a good confession."

I was one of the girls who helped Father Anselm get ready for Mass during retreat. I watched him in the sacristy of the chapel as he put on his vestments: first the amice, a square of white linen that covered his shoulders and symbolized a shield against the attacks of Satan; then the alb, a long white linen garment that reached to his feet and symbolized the innocence and purity necessary for the priest about to offer the holy sacrifice of the Mass; and then the chasuble, the outer vestment, shaped like a bell that symbolizes the yoke of unselfish service to the Lord. One morning he said to me, "Susan, we don't have any holy water." He handed me a silver bowl. "Get some water out of the tap."

I went over to the corner sink and filled the bowl and handed it to him. He made a hurried sign of the cross over it and mumbled something in Latin.

"There," he said. "Now it's holy water."

I had always thought that somehow holy water came from the Vatican . . . maybe in special vats, transported across the ocean from Rome to Connecticut.

In the spring of sophomore year, we had our first dance. The boys were bused in from Fairfield Prep, the Jesuit school. We wore nylon tulle dresses in pale, pastel colors over scratchy crinoline petticoats and little, flat ballerina shoes. We wore lengths of gauzy nylon tulle draped over our shoulders and over our "bosoms." The dance was held in the large wood-paneled foyer of the mansion. The nuns hung over the balcony that looked down on the foyer and clucked and fussed at us like a flock of agitated black and white penguins.

"Marie, may I see you please?"

"Yes, Sister."

"Marie, you're dancing too close to that boy. You have been reminded many times to keep the Holy Ghost between you."

"Yes, Sister."

At the end of my sophomore year, I made a sudden decision that I didn't understand myself. I tried out for the school play. It was to be a production of *Murder In a Nunnery*, a comic mystery, set in a convent school. The heroine of the play was a Spanish girl named Inez. I won the part. Rehearsals were held every day after school for six weeks. I loved every minute. I had discovered a fantasy world away from the suffocating world of the real convent school. I could transform myself into the spunky and funny character who spoke her mind, who didn't need the nuns to tell her how to solve the mystery, who said, "I know what I'm doing. I don't care what you all think. I can take care of myself!" Finally, opening night arrived. I was thrilled at the exhilaration of performing well, of being able to move the audience to laughter, then to suspense and back to laughter again. I was thrilled, too, that I could become someone other than "me." If I wasn't sure enough to speak my mind, the vivacious character I played was. And the audience loved that character . . . or was it me?

That summer, I made another sudden decision. I'd heard about the Westport Country Playhouse, a well-known summer stock theatre in Westport, Connecticut, just a few miles south of Fairfield. The theatre was owned by Laurence Langner, a co-founder of The Theatre Guild in New York, one of the most powerful and respected theatrical producing organizations in America. The Guild was known for its high artistic standards and the diverse selections of plays and musicals that it sent to Broadway. It had produced many successes, including the musical *Oklahoma* and others. The Westport Country Playhouse was one of a number of summer theatres in New England in those days called "the straw-hat circuit." The productions originated in New York, where the play was cast and directed, and then the plays went out "on the road." They stopped for a week at each of the summer theatres on the circuit.

I'd heard that the playhouse ran a summer apprentice program for college students who were studying for careers in the professional theatre. You had to be eighteen to be accepted as a summer apprentice. Without telling anyone, I got up at dawn one early summer morning, walked down to the Post Road and caught the bus for Westport. I was fifteen, but I was tall. I breathlessly told the managing director that I was eighteen and that I hadn't decided yet where I wanted to go to college but I wanted to become an actress and I wanted to study and learn everything I could about my chosen profession. He wouldn't be able to find a more dedicated student, I said. I had always loved the theatre, and since I came from a long line of performers and dancers, I wanted to carry on the family tradition and everyone at home would be so proud of me if I were accepted. I talked my way into the program. Then I took the bus back home and told my parents that I was now an apprentice at the playhouse. My mother had just had a new baby, my youngest brother, and she and my father were so busy and preoccupied with their infant son that they seemed relieved not to have to worry about how I would spend my summer. My mother agreed to drive me down to the playhouse every morning, and one of the staff members or older apprentices would drive me home at night.

The theatre was housed in an old, red barn at the end of a narrow, tree-shaded lane just off the Post Road in Westport. The stage and the rows of cushioned, wooden benches where the audience sat were on the second floor of the barn. Two sets of stairs, one stage right and the other left, led down to the ground floor and the greenroom or "greeting" room, where the actors received backstage visitors. Off the greenroom were the dressing rooms for the actors and the wardrobe room. A wide door, the backstage door, led from the greenroom out-side to a narrow alleyway that ran along the back of the barn and separated it from three other old wooden outbuildings, also painted red, that were once part of the original farmstead.

The first of these outbuildings faced the backstage door and was used for storing "props," the theatrical term for "properties" or the furniture and accessories used to decorate the stage. The building adjoining was the set designer's studio. The ceilings had been removed to create a high open space where the designer could paint the "flats" or the backdrops that were the settings, the background scenery, for the plays. The designer laid the flats, enormous canvasses stretched over wood frames, on the floor of his studio and walked around them, painting the canvasses with brushes attached to a long wooden handle. He painted blue skies with puffy white clouds or elaborate vistas of Italian gardens or ornate walls of French drawing rooms. When each new show came into the theatre, the new sets were carried across the alleyway and hoisted up through a high door over the backstage door onto the stage. There the master carpenter nailed them into place.

The last building of the three stood next to the lane that led out to the Post Road. This housed the administrative offices of the people who ran the business of the playhouse; the producers, the business manager, public relations director and the stage manager.

There were thirteen other apprentices in the program that sum-mer. Of course, I was the youngest. They were all college students or graduate students at the University of Pennsylvania, Princeton, Yale and Harvard, majoring in theatre arts, and preparing for careers in the professional theatre. One of the girls was British and had spent the summer before as an apprentice at the Old Vic, the Royal Victoria Theatre, in London, one of the most highly regarded theatres in Europe. One of the young men was also British, a student at Oxford. Another young man was an Israeli.

Every week, on Sunday afternoon, a new play came to the theatre with a new director and a new cast. Every week we were assigned a specific duty so we could learn every aspect of the business of presenting a play. The first week I was assigned to assist the costume designer and the wardrobe mistress. The play was *Anastasia*, about the mystery surrounding one of the young daughters of the murdered Czar Nicholas of Russia. The costumes were delivered to the backstage door on Sunday morning for dress rehearsal Sunday night and I helped the costume designer carry them in and hang them on the clothing racks in each dressing room. That afternoon I helped her fit the actors and actresses in long, full-skirted period dresses and gray swallow-tailed formal coats. I pinned up hems and helped her take in seams. I spent the days of that week in the wardrobe room, among the racks of brightly colored ball gowns and formal gray coats, carefully pressing the ladies' long, taffeta skirts and washing and ironing the men's white cotton shirts. At night before the curtain went up I laced the ladies into their corsets, helped them into hoop petticoats and long dresses and trailed after them up the stairs to the stage holding the dresses up off the ground and tilting their hoop skirts sideways to fit through the narrow stairwell.

One of the actresses was Lilly Darvas, a tall, rail-thin Hungarian woman of aristocratic bearing and older years. She had high cheekbones, pale translucent skin and silver-white hair worn swept back in a chignon. She spoke softly and carefully with a slight, indefinable European accent and she moved with the graceful elegance of someone used to being watched and admired. There was a trace of sadness in her deep-set brown eyes, as if something or someone precious to her had been irretrievably lost. Once, she had been a famous performer in her native land, but the war had ravaged her home and her culture. Now she was here, in Connecticut, in a converted barn, in the heat of a New England summer, playing a Dowager Empress in a play about another ruined country and family.

Every night when the curtain rang down I waited for her in the wings. She came off stage in a heavy black dress that was drenched in sweat. Her beautiful face was wet under the oily mask of grease-paint. The dress dragged heavily behind her as I helped her down the stairs into her dressing room. Only when she was inside with the door closed did she allow her shoulders to sag under the weight of the dress. I helped her struggle out of the thing that weighed almost as much as she. She sat slumped in her chair before the mirror with its rows of electric lights and fanned herself in the stifling summer heat. She reached for the jar of cold cream and box of Kleenex and slowly began to remove the heavy, flesh-colored greasepaint from her face and neck. Then she took a small, silver soap dish from the top of the dressing table, got up and crossed to the sink in the corner of the dressing room, and carefully washed her face and neck and arms. Then she sat down again in front of the lighted mirror and splashed a lightly fragranced perfume on her shoulders, neck and arms. This was the last part of the silent ritual, one that, it seemed to me, she had performed too many times to count. She sat back in the chair, closed her eyes and let out a long, deep sigh as if divesting herself of the last remnants of the character she'd played on the stage above. "There," she said. "It's over." She stared for a moment at her reflection in the mirror and then she murmured, "Adieu . . . until tomorrow." She reached for the bottle of perfume again and dabbed a single drop in the hollow of her throat. The fragrance held the faint sweet scent of lemon and jasmine . . . exotic, as if from some old and faraway European garden. "What is that perfume?" I asked. "It's beautiful."

"It's 'Arpege,' from the house of Lanvin."

"Lanvin?"

"Yes, my dear. La parfumerie. In Paris. You know."

"Oh," I said. I was dazzled.

The next morning I let myself into her dressing room. She had arranged her make-up carefully in a neat row on the dressing table next to her little silver soap dish and a silver hairbrush. A clean white washcloth and towel were folded on the shelf above the sink. The room still held the scent of her perfume. I took the black dress, which she'd placed carefully on a hanger on the clothing rack, and took it outside into the small, enclosed yard at the side of the theatre where I hung the men's shirts out to dry. I pinned the heavy dress to the clothesline in the shade so it wouldn't fade but would freshen in the breeze. Later in the day I returned it to her dressing room.

At the end of the last performance on Saturday night, I helped Miss Darvas down to her dressing room as usual. On this last night, she packed her things and made herself ready to move on with the show to the next theatre. She sat for the last time at her dressing table and then turned to me. She handed me a small box, beautifully wrapped in black and silver paper and tied with a silver ribbon. "This is for you, Susan, with my thanks," she said.

"Oh!" I said. "I haven't done anything at all."

"I dreaded wearing that black dress," she said. "Thank you for hanging it in the fresh air every day. It always smelled so sweet. Now open your gift."

Inside the box was a bottle of Arpege. I was overcome. "Thank you Miss Darvas," I said. "Whenever I wear this I'll think of you."

"No, my dear, think of the theatre," she said. "And I'll remember that you made it a pleasure for me to perform. That is everything for an actress."

We apprentices worked from nine in the morning straight through until eleven o'clock at night. After the curtain rang down and our jobs in the theatre were done for the night, we all went out together to Barna's, a restaurant just down the road from the playhouse. We sat and talked about the performances the actors had given and the choices the directors had made. We talked about books and plays and playwrights: Chekhov, Ibsen, Brecht, Weill, Williams, O'Neil,

Saroyan, Odets. My *Fair Lady* opened that summer, and we all knew the entire score by heart. Someone always sat down at the piano and launched into "On the Street Where You Live" or "Get Me to the Church on Time." I loved the world I found myself in. I loved every minute of it.

One week in the middle of the summer, I was assigned to assist Bill, the gruff, older, white-haired man who was the master carpenter. I would work with him until all the carpentry work was finished and the sets were complete. At night, I would help the stage manager clean up the greenroom and the dressing rooms after each performance. We were constructing the stage sets for a play that would star Tallulah Bankhead, a legendary American actress who'd been a star on Broadway in the forties but whose career, in this summer of 1956, was in decline. On the Sunday afternoon that her play came into the theatre, I was upstairs on the stage with Bill helping him construct a set of stairs that Miss Bankhead would use to make her entrance in the first act. The stairs were on their side as we worked on them. When they were finished he would right them and move them to center stage.

When the curtain rose she would be discovered standing on the top of the platform, in a long white dress, holding a cigarette in a long holder. She was to spread her arms wide to the audience and say "Dahlings!" and then come down these stairs that Bill and I were making to the stage. I'd seen the dress she would wear when the costume designer took it from the van with other costumes for the show. It was a shimmering, long, white satin column of a dress, and the costume designer carried it into Miss Bankhead's dressing room draped across her arms as if it were an offering, and hung it carefully, high off the floor, on the clothing rack.

Bill sent me down to the greenroom to get some tools. As I started down the dark, narrow stairway to the greenroom a woman lurched up the stairs, bumping me as she passed. She stumbled onto the stage.

I saw her stagger up to Bill who was kneeling next to the set of steps, still laying on its side. The woman looked down at him and then at the steps.

She walked around them, inspecting them, staggering up against them as she went. Suddenly she turned on Bill. "How can I possibly be expected to make an entrance down these fucking things! I won't use these! God damn you all! Make new ones!" Her voice was raw, husky.

Bill stood up. He was a tall man and he towered over her. "Who do you think you are?" he said. "There's a young girl here!" The woman turned then and stared at me as I stood, transfixed, at the top of the stairs. It was Tallulah Bankhead. She was in her early fifties, thin, haggard-looking. She had heavy-lidded eyes and straight, lank brown hair, and in the harsh glare of the carpenter's work light her skin looked pale, grayish and it sagged on her neck. She wore heavy, red lipstick and there were deep lines etched around her mouth. A cigarette dangled from her lips.

"Well, she better see what actresses expect! She's here to learn, right? Actresses expect the best!" Her voice was harsh, and her words were slurred, and ran together. She leaned on the stairs for support. "Make new ones! Now!"

"You'd better sleep it off or you won't come down any stairs," Bill said.

"I can't come down these! Look at them!"

Bill paused for a moment as if trying to control his temper. "Can't you see these stairs are laying on their side?" he asked quietly. "They'll be right-side-up when you make your entrance." She bent down and peered at them. Bill motioned to me over her shoulder. I went over to him.

"Get her off this stage. Bring her back down to her dressing room," he whispered.

"Miss Bankhead," I said. She rose unsteadily to her feet and glared at me.

"Let's go down to your dressing room," I said. "It's cooler down there and you can sit down."

"Fuck! What makes you think I want to sit down?" Tallulah Bankhead was the first person I'd ever heard use that word. I had no idea what it meant. Her face had turned a deep red. She plucked the cigarette out of her mouth and flicked it on the floor toward my feet. I picked it up, instantly. I was horrified. You never defiled the stage—and think of the fire hazard!

"I won't have some green kid telling me what to do!"

By now, Bill had heard and seen enough. "She didn't tell you what to do. She's trying to help you."

"I don't need help from some cute young thing!"

He took her by one arm and propelled her off the stage into the wings. I could hear her ranting at him as he took her back down the stairs into the greenroom. But all I could think of was the still-smoking cigarette butt in my hand. I went over to Bill's work table and doused it in an empty coffee cup. Bill came back up onto the stage. "Stay away from her," he said. "There's nothing you can learn from her."

After the opening night performance Miss Bankhead was the last to leave. Finally she swept out with a group of friends, and I went into her dressing room to clean it. I smelled dank sweat, spilled whiskey and stale cigarette smoke. I saw open jars of make-up, dirty glasses and overflowing ashtrays strewn across the top of her dressing table. The cigarette butts were smeared with lipstick. Clumps of used Kleenex and more cigarette butts littered the floor. The shimmering white satin dress was on the floor where she had stepped out of it.

The costume designer came in behind me. I watched her pick up the costume and hold it up to examine it. The white satin was stained with sweat and dirt from the dressing room floor. The designer shook her head in disgust and looked around the room. "What a shame," she said. She went over to the wastebasket under the dressing table and picked an empty whiskey bottle out of it. She shook her head again and sighed and dropped the empty bottle back into the basket.

Just before the curtain went up for the last show of that week a rumor flashed down to the greenroom from the box office. Elizabeth Taylor and her husband, Mike Todd, were in the audience! The apprentices who were ushering had seen her! The apprentices working high on the light bridge over the audience had seen her! We were stuck backstage. . . . When could we see her? Would we see her? What if we missed her? And then came wonderful news. She was coming backstage after the show to see Miss Bankhead!

When the curtain finally rang down we waited breathlessly in a corner of the greenroom. Suddenly, in the alley outside, a dense crowd of people appeared, moving as one, flowing toward the greenroom door. Just at the door, as if by some miracle, the crowd parted for a single moment, and I saw her, the young star, already a legendary beauty, and her husband. They were unbelievably small! The crowd around them seemed to tower over them. She was short, curvacious and deeply tanned and she wore a white scooped-neck summer dress, cinched at the waist with a rose-colored belt. Her jet-black hair fell to her shoulders and her violet eyes were gentle, luminous. Her husband wore a tan suit and a white shirt open at the neck. He was only as tall as she, but slight, wiry, with sandy-colored hair, sharp features and light blue eyes that were watchful, wary. As suddenly as the crowd around them had parted, it began to close in on them again, and in that instant I saw her violet eyes grow wide, frightened. A look of panic crossed her beautiful face, and we saw her husband put his forearm out in front of her as if to block the crowd, keep it away from her. But the crowd couldn't seem to stay away. Arms and hands reached toward her as if trying to take some of her gentle beauty. She was trapped, helpless, until her husband turned, caught her by the arm and darted with her out the door they had just come through. The last glimpse I had of her was of her terror-stricken face as she fled the crowd that adored her.

Where could she ever go that she would not be known? Could she ever be safe alone? Could she ever believe that the people she met wanted to know her and not the movie star? Was that the price of fame? It was the first time I ever realized that "appearance" has a human cost.

One week the young John Cassavetes and his wife, Gena Rowlands came to the playhouse in a production called *Three by Tennessee*, three one-act plays by Tennessee Williams. They were a striking couple. He was small, darkly handsome, with a sharp nose and intense brown eyes. She was in her early twenties, taller than he, a graceful, winsome blonde. The production also starred Maureen Stapleton, an edgy, high-strung woman in her thirties with dyed red hair, small blue eyes and the thick features of an Irish peasant. The other player was an older character actor named Jules Munshin. Julie, as we were allowed to call him, was an endearing, burly man in his forties with a round face, soulful brown eyes and dark thinning hair. He was a veteran of vaudeville, the theatre and movies and had appeared with Frank Sinatra and Gene Kelly in the movie musical *On the Town*.

I was assigned to the property mistress, Laraine. The week before the show came in, I went out with her into Westport and the surrounding towns to gather stage furniture and props. We went to antique stores and junk shops, and we raided the attics of loyal audience members who'd volunteered to loan us whatever we needed for the show. We hauled everything back in an old pickup truck and stored our finds in the prop "room," the wooden building next to the set designer's studio. The three-room building was already crammed with old furniture, clocks, oriental rugs, overstuffed sofas and elaborately carved wooden writing desks. At the very front, tucked into a space next to Laraine's desk, was an old mahogany harpsichord and a Victorian side chair with a plush red velvet seat and curved, gilt-edged legs. Opposite her desk, in glass cases, were sets of old sterling silverware, enameled hand mirrors, embroidered ladies fans and beaded purses, men's gold pocket watches and ivory-handled walking sticks. There was a pink feather boa and a pair of men's spats.

When the show came in, the property mistress and set designer and director worked together to "set" the stage, and I worked backstage during performances to make sure the actors had their personal props.

I'd noticed in rehearsal that Mr. Cassavetes was impatient with any disruption or delay. On opening night, thinking I could save him some time before the performance, I offered to check his props for him. "No!" he said, abruptly. Then he caught himself and smiled at me. He softened his tone. "A good actor always gets to the theatre two hours before the curtain goes up to check his own props and costumes. When I walk out on stage I want to know everything is in place. That way I'm in control. When I know everything's in order, I'm free to give my best performance. Remember that, honey."

On opening night I noticed that all but one of the actors arrived two hours before the curtain went up at 8:30. They checked their costumes and props in their dressing rooms and then went upstairs to the stage and made sure that every prop they needed was in its place either on stage or off stage.

Only one actor didn't check his props. He arrived late, a half hour before the curtain was to go up, and he came into the greenroom in a great flurry, demanding to know if his costume had been pressed. I heard Miss Rowlands remark to her husband, "I wish he'd be more considerate. He's making everyone nervous." After the show, he drew more attention to himself in the greenroom, talking loudly, still wearing his costume and make-up. Several other apprentices stood with me, watching the man make a production of himself. I saw Julie

Munshin sitting quietly at his dressing table, looking at the man through the open door of his dressing room. He saw us and motioned us into his dressing room. "Acting is a profession, kids," he said. "It isn't a lifestyle. It's a job. A good actor gets to the theatre on time and plays a character for a few hours. When the play is over, he takes his make-up off and hangs up his costume. Then he goes home. The character stays at the theatre."

My sixteenth birthday fell at the end of that week. After the Friday night show, we'd planned to meet, as usual, at Barna's. The prop mistress and I and several other apprentices were just leaving the greenroom when Julie asked me to stay behind to help him find a prop he said he'd misplaced. We went upstairs to look for it, a gold pocket watch with a chain. Julie was a meticulous performer, and I remember thinking how odd it was for him to lose a personal prop. Upstairs, the theatre was dark except for the work lights above the stage. Julie rattled around backstage, talking to himself as he moved behind the sets. I stood for a moment on the apron of the stage and looked out into the darkness of the theatre. It was a familiar darkness to me, warm, comforting. I remember wondering if I would ever feel safer than I did at that moment. Julie came up to stand beside me. "It's something, isn't it," he said. He swept his hand out toward the darkness. "We actors give gifts. Every performance is a gift." Then he took a step back and made a deep bow to the invisible audience. Then he turned to me. "Come on, little one," he said. "Time to go."

"Did you find your prop?" I said.

"Oh," he said. "I think I did leave it on my dressing table where it belongs. Come on, we'll drive down to the restaurant." As we pulled into the parking lot, the lights were on inside, but no one was sitting at the tables.

"Julie," I said. "There isn't anyone there."

"Oh?" he said, and opened his brown eyes very wide as if shocked. "Well, we'll go in and wait for them."

We went in and sat down at one of the empty tables. Suddenly people appeared from every hidden corner of the place. "Surprise!" they screamed. "Susie! Surprise!" Julie looked at me. He was beaming. "How could you turn sixteen and not have a celebration?"

"You didn't lose your prop after all, did you?" I said.

"Of course not! Mazel tov!"

My parents didn't mind the late hours I kept. Many nights when I came home, my mother was up waiting for me, sitting in her rocking chair, cradling my little brother, feeding him while she watched the *Late Show* or the Steve Allen show on T.V. In those times, late at night, I thought I saw a look of longing cross her face when I told her about the wonderful new people I was meeting and the exciting work I was learning to love.

Sometimes we apprentices went along into New York with the older staff members of the playhouse and watched shows in rehearsal in studios near Broadway. We'd go out afterwards with the actors to Downey's Restaurant on Eighth Avenue. We ate corned beef sandwiches and drank iced tea and listened to the actors talk about the value of good, solid training in the theatre, the importance of technique and originality in acting, and the necessity of study in dance for movement and voice lessons for vocal range and versatility. "Think of your body and your voice as instruments of your craft," they would say. "It is essential to imagine and study and practice all the time if you want to be an actor. Discipline yourself!" We listened raptly and believed.

We'd leave the restaurant and walk along Broadway, just as crowds were gathering under the glittering marquees. You could see the ladies and gentlemen inside in the lobbies of the theatres, standing in small groups, laughing, talking, anticipating, waiting to be transported, waiting for the make-believe to begin. I loved the theatre. I loved New York and Broadway. It was a world of fantasy but of order and discipline, as well. It was where I wanted to spend the rest of my life. I knew that. I was sixteen.

Toward the end of the summer the managing director of the play-house called me to his office. He told me that I would be assistant to the stage manager for the last play of the summer season. To be named assistant to the stage manager was an honor and a great responsibility because the stage manager is responsible for every aspect of the play as it is being performed. The stage manager goes to the door of each actor's dressing room and calls the time before the curtain goes up: "Half hour, ladies and gentlemen," "Fifteen min-utes," "Five minutes." And finally, just before the curtain is to rise, "Places, please," and the actors leave their dressing rooms and take their places on the darkened stage behind the curtain. The stage manager calls for the house lights to dim, the stage lights to come up and then gives the cue for the curtain to rise. I couldn't believe at first that I'd been chosen for this privilege. I was thrilled. The play would star Sid Ceasar and Imogene Coca, the reigning comedy pair of the day. Julie Munshin would be a featured player in the cast.

On opening night the stage manager and I sat on high stools in the wings off stage right. I sat right next to him with a copy of the script in my lap and a flashlight and followed each line of dialogue. The stage manager called light cues and sound cues into his small intercom as the play progressed. Finally, the curtain rang down and then rose again for the actors to take their curtain calls. Mr. Ceasar and Miss Coca left the stage, but Julie stayed behind. He walked downstage to the footlights and addressed the audience. "I want to introduce you to one of the young people who help keep this theatre of ours alive. She's only a girl, but she's so dedicated! She loves every part of theatre. Susie! Susie!" I sat there on my assistant stage man-ager's stool completely confused. This was certainly not in the script. Who was he calling to? Julie rushed across the stage to where I sat in the wings. He plucked me off my stool and led me by the hand to the center of the stage, where I stood, dumfounded, in my T-shirt, dungaree shorts and sneakers. "This is our Susie," he said to the audience. "Isn't she adorable?"

I couldn't think of anything to say. I shrugged my shoulders and smiled. The audience roared. I could see my friends, fellow apprentices, in the wings, clapping and cheering. The stage manager was beaming. I couldn't understand any of it. All I knew was that I loved the work. And the approval.

I spent one day at home that entire summer. I had a dentist's appointment in the late morning and afterward I went down to the beach with Pepper. She loved to swim, and I hadn't spent much time with her all summer. She trotted ahead of me and made a beeline for the water. A group of girls I knew from Lauralton was gathered around the refreshment stand at the top of the beach. I went over to say hello.

"Susan!" called one. "You've got even skinnier!"

It was true, I had. I never thought about food until I was famished and even then had little time to eat. The girls wore two-piece bathing suits, make-up, lipstick and hairspray. They were sweating in the sun. They were talking about their boyfriends, football players from Fairfield Prep, and about weekend trips over the state line into Portchester, New York, where they drank beer.

"What have you been doing all summer?" asked one.

"I've been apprenticing at the Westport Country Playhouse," I said.

"What's an apprentice?"

"You learn all about the theatre."

"Oh," she said. "That's right. You were so good as Inez."

"Are there any cute boys there?" asked another.

"They're not really boys," I said. "They're all in college."

"Are you going out with one?"

"We all go out," I said. "We all go into New York, or out after the shows."

"Oh!" they cried. "You go to Portchester? We were in Portchester on Saturday night. John Lynch and Eddie Fahey got so drunk they both threw up in Paul Redgate's car! God! It got all over our skirts!"

On the last weekend of the season, the playhouse producers held an apprentice showcase. They invited every agent and producer and director who could come from New York to see us perform. We were to act in short scenes that we had either written or taken from other plays. One of the apprentices, a young man from Princeton, asked me to do a scene with him for the showcase. He'd adapted our scene from a short story by J. D. Salinger called "Just Before the War With the Eskimos" in which a troubled and eccentric young man named Franklin meets a much younger, innocent, teen-aged friend of his sister's named Ginnie. Ginnie is puzzled at Franklin's eccentricities, but she's a sympathetic listener. She thinks Franklin is crazy. But she feels sorry for him. It becomes clear that the young girl is more mature than the older man. We rehearsed the scene for days.

There was not an empty seat in the playhouse on the night of the apprentice showcase. Seven scenes were to be presented. We were to go on next to the last. I never had stage fright. I just couldn't wait to get on stage, and once on, I lost myself in the part. As the curtain rang down on our scene the audience applauded wildly. They cheered and whistled. Again, I could not understand why.

After the showcase, the greenroom downstairs was filled with people. They crowded around me, and in my great excitement I couldn't remember their names. I knew only that I'd entertained them. Somehow I had delighted them. It was the most wonderful thing I could think of to do. I thought I would never do anything else. I wanted to spend the rest of my life in the theatre.

One afternoon, a month or so after school had started again in the fall, my mother picked me up from the train station. She sat waiting for me in the car. She looked distressed.

"What's the matter?" I said.

"There's something I should have told you," she said. "This came for you." She handed me a letter addressed to me in the care of my parents.

"It's addressed to me," I said. "Why did you open it?"

"I thought it was to Dad and me," she said. "But it was for you."

"Dear Susan," I read. "I can't tell you how much I enjoyed your performance last Saturday night at the playhouse. Could you come in to see me as soon as possible? A role has come up that we think you would be perfect for. The producers of the play saw you on Saturday night and asked me to contact you. Rehearsals will be starting soon. You are quite a talented young lady. Please call me as soon as possible." A woman, an agent at the William Morris Agency, had signed it.

"When did this come?" I said.

"Three weeks ago," she said. I was stunned. I felt as though someone had hit me in the stomach.

"Why didn't you tell me?" I said, breathlessly. "Why didn't you give this to me when it came? How could you have done this to me?" Now I was incensed. My mother looked at me, shocked, and she began to stutter.

"We didn't want you to leave school," she said. "We talked to the agent, and she said you'd have to leave school. Dad didn't want you to leave school. You would have had a tutor, but Dad didn't want you to go to New York. I said you could have stayed with your grandmother, but he didn't want you to leave school."

"Why do you keep saying that? Stop talking about school!" I cried out. "Why did you keep this from me? Why didn't you tell me?"

My mother stammered, "I . . . I . . . We . . ." I hated to see her stutter. I tried to soften my words.

"Why, Mom? Didn't you know how important this was to me?"

She didn't answer me. After a long moment she said, "Isn't it wonderful that she thinks you're so talented?"

We drove home in silence. I went into the house and called the number the woman had written in the letter.

"Oh, yes," she said. "Susan. How nice to hear from you, dear. I spoke with your parents several weeks ago. We needed their permission for you to come meet the producers, but they said no. Didn't they tell you?"

"No," I said. "My mother just gave me your letter."

"Oh," she said. "I see. Well, the role the producers wanted you to take was filled by someone else. But the next time you're in New York, stop by."

At Lauralton, I waited to graduate. The last two years were stifling, stupefying. In senior year, we were required to take a theology class. The school chaplain, a priest who lived on the grounds with two perfectly matched black-and-white cocker spaniels, taught the class. One day he discussed a gospel in which Christ told his apostles that in heaven their happiness would be complete. The apostles would be happier than ordinary people, the priest said, in the same way that he and the nuns would be happier than laypeople.

"Our cups shall run over," said the priest. I raised my hand.

"Yes, Susan," he said. He looked resigned.

"If each one of us will be completely happy in heaven, then priests and nuns can't be happier than we'll be, Father."

"Yes, they can, Susan."

"Why?"

"Our cups are bigger," he said.

There was a snort from the back of the room.

"Isn't that right, Miss Reynolds?"

"I guess so, Father," said Joan.

I raised my hand again. He glared at me.

"Yes, Susan?"

"We're all servants of God," I said. For some reason I felt cheated, angry. "Why should you be happier than I? Then heaven wouldn't be heaven because there we would find comparisons. Comparisons don't make any one very happy."

"The gospel is the truth."

"I don't believe it."

I spent more and more time in Guidance with Sister Denise.

"Susan, why do you disagree with Father?" she said.

"Because . . . I don't think we have to be nuns or priests to be happy in heaven."

"Why do you constantly question?"

"I'm not questioning, Sister," I said. "I don't believe what he says." She put her hand to her forehead, closed her eyes and changed the subject.

"Won't you at least think of entering the convent?"

"No, Sister. I keep telling you that."

"But it would be such a worthy sacrifice for you to make. Remember that we sacrifice ourselves in this life so that we can be happy with Christ in the next."

"No! I can't give my life up like that!" I began to cry.

"Well, then what do you want to do?"

I couldn't answer her. But I couldn't stop crying.

"Well?"

"It doesn't matter!" .

"Susan, you're overwrought. You'll make everyone else upset. Think of others. Try to control yourself."

But I was losing control. I'd lost the theatre . . . what I'd lived for . . . what I relied on. The theatre was the place where I could put on a "persona" or "mask," assume a role and become someone, anyone, who mattered . . . someone who others liked, approved of, accepted. When the promise of the theatre was lost, I was left to fall back on myself—and there was no "self" there.

I went into New York almost every weekend to see my friends from the playhouse. Sometimes in my rush to get away from the school I took the train on Friday afternoon still wearing my school uniform. I changed my clothes in the ladies room of Grand Central Station. I put on nylon stockings, high heels, a black straight skirt and a black sweater with the sleeves pushed up. I tied a small, red silk scarf around my neck and put on the black beret that my Aunt Lucille had bought for me in Paris. I never wore the beret in Fairfield. In Fairfield, you only wore a hat on Sunday, to church. Then you wore a straw hat trimmed with fabric flowers in summer, or you wore a black lace veil. You never wore a beret in Fairfield. If you did, people might say you were a "bohemian."

I walked through Grand Central Station and met my friends from the playhouse under the Biltmore Hotel clock, and then we'd go out to dinner. After dinner, we'd go up to the Rainbow Room at the top of the RCA building to dance. We sat at the small tables that ringed the dance floor and smoked French cigarettes. My friends ordered champagne cocktails and whiskey sours. I was still too young to be served alcohol, so I ordered ginger ale. Many weekend nights we went over to Radio City Music Hall to see a movie or to Broadway to see a play. But I never went to meet the agent.

Many of my friends had graduated from college and were living in their own apartments in the city, doing what all young actors do in New York—hoping and dreaming of "making it"—but I found that I had less and less in common with them. After that summer and the letter, the theatre was never the same. I never thought of it again as full of promise. The world I had loved was unattainable to me. It was closed. Finished. Stopped. I didn't understand why the loss of it filled me with such grief.

After my friends and I had danced, and they had gone back to their apartments and their dreams, I left Broadway and walked up Fifth Avenue by myself. In those days, in 1957, New York was a lovely, gleaming city. The sidewalks were fresh and scrubbed, and they shone under the streetlights. I walked through Rockefeller Plaza past the pools and the softly splashing fountains to Fifth Avenue. I passed the windows of Saks Fifth Avenue where, even late at night, the air was heavy with the perfume sold inside. I walked on up Fifth Avenue, past the sparkling windows of Tiffany's and the Steuben Glass Company. I watched doormen in gray uniforms and red hats polishing the brass fittings of the carved, wooden front doors of the old buildings on Fifth Avenue, and I watched as they swept the carpets that lay under the awnings that stretched from the front doors to the street. I walked all the way up to the Plaza Hotel at Central Park just to see the long line of black hansom cabs with their drivers, sitting up in their high seats, waiting in front of the hotel for passengers to drive through the park. Then I walked back to Fifty-ninth Street and turned the corner to wait for the bus to Queens and my Grandmother Ryan's house. When I was sixteen and seventeen and eighteen, I could walk from Broadway to the East side and up Fifth Avenue, alone at night with no fear at all, in this city that I'd once thought would be my home.

I got on the bus and it crossed the East River, far over Welfare Island and the hospitals below, back to Queens. No matter how quietly I let myself in, my grandmother always heard me and called to me. "Sleep well, dear."

"Thank you, Gram. You, too."

But very late at night the soft chimes of the grandfather's clock would wake me. It had been her wedding present, and it still stood in the hallway outside the bedrooms. My grandfather had listened to it strike the hours and the quarter hours of the last days of his life. Maybe the soft chimes reminded him of his quiet days in the seminary before he emerged into the real world of unexpected circumstance and lost promise. I went down into the kitchen, unable to sleep. She woke then, too, and came into the kitchen. She poured milk into a copper pan and lit the stove. She put out the old blue and white china cups and saucers that had been her mother's, and then filled them with the warm milk. She sat down across from me at the kitchen table and reached for my hand.

"What is done is done. You must not let the past overwhelm you."

"I know."

"Think ahead, my dear girl. Always think ahead."

"Yes, Gram."

"Remember, you always have yourself."

How could she have known that I had lost that?

CHAPTER ELEVEN

Appearances

I always wore my school uniform when I took the train back to Fairfield after those weekends in New York. One Sunday afternoon just before I graduated from Lauralton Hall, I got a ride to Fairfield with my friend Jessie, who was going through to New Haven to visit her parents. We met for breakfast in the city and then drove up to Connecticut. We wore our high heels and nylon stockings, straight, black skirts and tight, black turtleneck sweaters. We had short, pixie haircuts. Jessie wore small, gold hoop earrings and I wore my black beret. We'd seen Leslie Caron and Gene Kelly in *An American in Paris* and we'd decided to be very "French." We were still intoxicated with the Gershwin songs and spectacular dancing in the movie. The music always reminded me of my aunts dancing in my grandmother's kitchen when I was a little girl.

Before Jessie dropped me off at home, we stopped at the Fairfield Diner on the Post Road for coffee. Two men were sitting at the counter across from the door. One of them elbowed the man to his right. The other man turned to look at us over his shoulder. He gave a long, low whistle. We walked by them and slid into a booth near the back. Two older couples were sitting in the booth across the aisle from us. I recognized the women as friends of my mother's. I waved and smiled. The women nodded back at me, their lips in tight lines. They gave Jessie a long, cool, appraising look. The men didn't look at me or my friend. They sat with their arms crossed tightly in front of them and stared down at the table top. The women turned away and resumed their conversation.

"Who are those women?" asked Jessie.

"Friends of my mother's. She's in the Saint Thomas' Ladies Guild with them," I said.

"Oh," she said. "Is that the Catholic church?"

"Yes," I said. "We're Catholics. All my mother's friends are Catholics." She looked at me and raised her eyebrows.

"What's wrong?" I said.

"I don't know," she said. "Maybe they don't like people who look different." She gave a small laugh and shook her head. "Anyone who looks different must be a stranger in this town," she said.

"But I'm not a stranger," I said. "I live here. Those are my mother's friends!"

"You're a stranger. You just don't know it."

Jessie dropped me off at home and went on her way to New Haven. My father was sitting in the living room as I walked in. He looked up at me.

"What kind of a get-up is that?" he said.

"What?"

"What does your grandmother think of that outfit?"

"She says it looks quite smart," I said. "She made the skirt for me."

My father looked me up and down . . . at my black beret, my tight black turtleneck sweater, my black, slit skirt and my high heels. He folded his paper and got up from his chair. He went to the door of the living room and turned and looked at me again. He shook his head. Then he turned and went upstairs. I went out to the kitchen where my mother was making dinner and feeding my small brother in his highchair.

"You look so sophisticated!" said my mother. "Is that what they're wearing now in New York?"

"Yes," I said.

She picked me up at the train station the next day after school.

"Joan Campbell called me this morning," she said. "She saw you in the diner yesterday afternoon."

"Yes," I said. "She was there with her husband and the Gardners."

"Did you talk to them? Did you say hello?"

"I waved," I said. "Why?"

"She wondered where you were going dressed like that."

"Dressed like what?" I said. "What are you talking about?"

"Don't get so upset," she said. "I want you to know what she said."

"For heaven's sake," I said. "What did she say?"

"She said you and your friend looked fast."

"Fast?"

"Yes, like a tramp. Your father agreed. How many times have we told you that the way you look is a reflection on us? And that you're known by the company you keep?"

"Why do you say that?" I said. "Yesterday you told me how sophisticated I looked!"

"Oh," said my mother. "I said *what*?"

"Nothing."

My mother and father had always been surrounded by their own families, by people whose expectations they understood. They had moved to a new town and, for the first time in their lives, found themselves alone. They were "outsiders" in Fairfield. The only place of refuge for them, where they could be accepted and protected, was in the church and in a small circle of Catholic friends whose rules of conduct were the same. My parents never socialized with Protestants or Jews because they might not have been accepted by those people. As it was, it had taken several years for my mother to make friends within our Catholic parish. My mother was terrified of their disapproval—a lesson learned from her father. She never forgot his last words to her, "The only thing I had to leave you was my good name." My mother's reputation was the bedrock of her life.

I graduated from Lauralton Hall the next spring. That summer my father got me a job in the mail room at the Bridgeport Brass Company, where he was now the advertising manager. Most mornings I rode in to work with him. He'd never been interested in too much conversation, but it was a short ride so the silences weren't that awkward. One day, Ralph, the man in charge of the mailroom, told me to go to lunch early. I went into the cafeteria and saw my father, sitting alone at a table, having his lunch. I went over to him and leaned down and kissed his cheek. He instantly recoiled.

"What are you doing? Don't do that!"

"What?" I said. I went to sit down.

"No! Don't sit here!"

"Dad! What's the matter?"

"I don't want people to get the wrong idea. People don't know you work here. They'll think I'm meeting some beauty for lunch."

I got up, mortified, and went over to an empty table at the far end of the room. I sat down and started to eat my lunch by myself. I saw some of my father's friends sit down with him and begin their lunch. None of them noticed me, and my father didn't look my way, but I felt my face burning. I got up quietly, gathered my lunch bag and my pocketbook and left the cafeteria. I went back upstairs to the empty mail room and took the sandwich out of the lunch bag, but I couldn't eat it. I threw it away untouched.

I left Fairfield in September for Boston University, where I'd been accepted into the School of Fine and Applied Arts. I had meant to major in theatre arts. I went to classes in speech, dance, mime, acting and history of theatre. Although I tried to be interested in my classes, I couldn't summon any enthusiasm for any of them.

One Friday night, soon after I started college, I went over to Cambridge with two of my new friends from school. One of the girls, Sarah, had her own car, a small, old, Alfa Romeo. They had heard about a "mixer," a dance at one of the senior dormitories at Harvard. We drove across the Charles River and into Harvard Square. We found the dorm and went in. Inside, in the darkened dining hall, chairs and tables had been moved back and a band was playing a languorous, rhythmic ballad by Sam Cooke. "You send me . . . Darling, you send me . . . honest you do . . ." On the dimly lit dance floor, couples, young men and women, were dancing together, holding each other closely, swaying slowly, barely moving. The young men wore tweed jackets, Oxford cloth button-down shirts and thin, striped ties. They wore khaki trousers and wing-tip, cordovan shoes. The young women wore plaid, pleated skirts, Shetland wool cardigan sweaters and penny loafers.

The three of us were theatre students. We dressed entirely in black. I wore the black tights and ballet slippers that I put on for dance class with my black straight skirt, a wide, black leather belt and a black turtleneck sweater. I wore my black beret. As soon as we walked in, four or five young men came over to us. They were all Harvard seniors, easygoing, gracious, very sure of themselves. They weren't at all like the young, eager freshman boys over at Boston U. One of them, a handsome, tall blond with piercing blue eyes, asked me to dance. Soon, other young men began to cut in, and I was dancing every dance—the Lindy and the foxtrot and even the rumba— until I was breathless. But the tall blond asked me for every dance first. His name was Bob. He was a scholarship student at Harvard and on the swimming team. He was studying to be an engineer.

I told him where I went to school and my name, but nothing else. During the last slow dance he held me closer to him, and he bent down and whispered the words to the song in my ear, "Goodnight, sweetheart, till we meet tomorrow. Goodnight, sweetheart . . ." My breasts were pressed against him, and I thought that I should move a little away from him but I felt excited by the closeness. My head was close against his chest, and I felt my face begin to flush. I saw my friends waving at me from the door. I moved away from him and looked up at him.

"I have to leave," I said. "Our curfew is eleven o'clock."

"You have the sexiest eyes I've ever seen," he said.

"Thank you," I said. I felt my face grow even hotter. "I really do have to leave." I pulled away from him and went over to my friends at the door.

"Wait a minute," he called after me. "Give me your number!"

"Wow," said one of my friends. "He's really cute."

"Yeah," said the other. "And he was all over you."

I felt embarrassed. "Let's go," I said.

We went out and walked down the street to the car. It sat next to the curb looking strangely lopsided. One of the tires had gone completely flat. As we were rummaging around in the trunk looking for a jack, the tall blond young man from the dance and his three roommates came walking quickly up behind us.

"We have a flat tire and no jack," said Sarah.

"Lucky for me," said the blond, smiling over at me.

"This is a very tiny car," said one of his friends. "Ready, gentlemen?" Laughing, they tipped the car up on one side.

"Where's your lug wrench?" asked one, out of breath.

"What?" said Sarah. "What did you call me?"

"Wrench! Wrench!" they hooted.

They were finding this hilarious. One poked around again in the trunk, finding the wrench and the spare tire. Within minutes they had changed the tire and righted the little car.

"Now," said the tall blond to me. "Give me your phone number."

When we got back to the dormitory, the phone was ringing.

"Susan, it's for you," said Sarah.

He was calling to make sure we had arrived safely. Would I go out with him next weekend? I hesitated. I remembered how closely he had held me while we were dancing and how insistent he was when he asked for my phone number. I was uneasy about seeing him again. But then I remembered how smoothly he had danced with me. I remembered the feeling of my breasts pressed hard against his chest. He had told me I was beautiful, desirable. I agreed to see him the next Friday night.

He called for me at my dormitory, and we drove over to Harvard Square. We went to a movie and then to a small restaurant for hamburgers where we sat and talked about our hometowns and the courses we were taking. This night he didn't hold my hand or put his arm around me. We walked back to his car and drove across the river, back into Boston. He parked the car down the street from the dorm and as I moved to get out of the car he took my hand.

"Do you know how hard it is for me not to touch you?" he said. He leaned toward me. "Please kiss me," he said.

He took my face between his hands and began to kiss me on my mouth, hesitantly at first, and then softly and slowly until I opened my mouth under his. He moved his hands down to my neck and my shoulders and then he ran them lightly down my arms. He took my hands in his and bent and kissed them.

"I haven't been able to get you out of my mind," he said. "All I could think of was kissing you like this."

He drew me to him and kissed me . . . long, deep kisses again and again. Then he moved his hands down to my breasts. He cupped them in his hands.

"These are so beautiful," he whispered.

I pushed him away and crossed my arms over my breasts.

"No," I said. "No. I hardly know you. No."

"I'm sorry," he said. "I guess I'm moving too fast. But you are such a beautiful girl. I can't keep my hands off you. Please forgive me. Go out with me tomorrow?"

"No," I said. "This is really too much for me. I have to go in." And I got out of the car and walked quickly into the dorm.

All the dates I'd ever had were with young men I'd met in the theatre, older than myself like this man, but I'd gone out with them in groups with other friends. On the rare occasions when I did go out alone with a man, I behaved exactly as I'd been taught as a young Catholic woman. You never allowed a man to touch your breasts. You never allowed a man to kiss you passionately. Oh, I allowed someone's arm around my shoulders, perhaps even a modest kiss at the end of an evening, but I'd never met anyone who aroused me as sexually and as powerfully as this man did. I avoided his calls for the next several weeks because he made me uncomfortable and frightened. He made me want sex.

To have sex outside of marriage was to commit a mortal sin. All Catholics were taught that the primary purpose of sex was to create new life. Sex was not something that could be enjoyed for its own sake. And a Catholic woman was forbidden to use a contraceptive. I'd never had sex with a man. Suddenly, sex was enthralling to think about. But every time I thought about it I remembered the nuns' warnings and the frightening complications they said might follow it.

I was becoming aware of a strange, new power of my own. I knew I attracted men. They gazed at me. They wanted to be near me. They wanted to touch me. Now I knew I could use the power I had to attract men to fill my own need to be noticed, to be desired. I had no other sense of power or strength. If they thought I was beautiful, then I was. If they thought I was worthwhile, then I would be someone who mattered; I might even be lovable. I'd begun to depend on external things—appearances. My appearance. I didn't believe I had anything else to offer.

I spent every weekend of the first month at school going to more dances, more mixers, more parties. My grades began to slide. I couldn't forget the tall, blond, Harvard senior. The next time he called I talked to him. He invited me to the Saturday football game and the dance afterward.

He picked me up early, and we drove over to his dormitory where the young men were allowed to have girls visit them in their rooms on Saturdays, before and after the football games. We spent the two hours before the game alone in his room. He wondered why I had refused his phone calls. I tried to explain my fear of pregnancy to him. I tried to explain my beliefs . . . that I would go to hell if I were to have sex with him.

"Well, then we won't do that," he said. "But I can kiss you, can't I?"

"Oh, yes," I said. "Yes, you can."

I reached up and pulled him down to me and kissed him. I wanted to feel his tongue in my mouth again.

At the game, he put his arm around me. I couldn't stop touching him. I laid my hand on his leg, my head on his shoulder. I touched his face. On the way back to his room, we walked arm in arm. Several times he stopped and pulled me close to him and kissed me. Alone in his room, we sat down together on his bed, and as he kissed me, he slowly unbuttoned my blouse and took it off. He reached behind me and unhooked my bra and it fell away. He moved the palms of his hands softly over my breasts, cupped them and put his face between them and kissed them. Then he laid me down on the bed. He lay down next to me and slid one hand under my back. With the other he traced a line with his fingers from the hollow of my throat, down between my breasts, down my stomach and then put his fingers between my legs.

"No!" I gasped. "No!"

But I made no move to stop him. He found my sex and at the very moment that he touched it, lightly, a great wave of rapture rose up and rushed over me. The wave lifted me and carried me, helpless and willing, as it swelled, then crested and fell, and then swelled again. I heard myself moan and cry out. I heard the sound of bells ringing in my ears.

"The phone!" I gasped. "That's your phone!"

"What?"

"Don't you hear those bells ringing?" I said.

"I guess that was a good one," he said.

"That was my first one," I said.

I closed my eyes and sighed, and as I did, the pale moonlike face of Sister Denise rose up before me, placid and serene, encased in her white wimple. I sat upright.

"Oh, my God," I said. "So this is why she wanted us to join the convent." But, I wondered, how did she know?

I saw Bob every weekend for the next month. We went to football games and parties and dances. The extra hours that we spent in his room were sensual and exciting, but I would not give in completely to the desire he aroused in me. He wondered why I would not touch him. I didn't tell him that I was afraid that if I did, I wouldn't be able to restrain him, that he would enter me and I would lose control over anything that might happen next.

He tried to persuade me to touch him, but I resisted. He began to argue with me. Why couldn't I think of him? He would protect us. Didn't I trust him? He became more and more insistent. I began to feel guilty. But still I resisted.

He started to be angry on many of those Saturday afternoons. How could I believe that sex between us was a sin when I had gone this far? This was not fair to him. I wasn't being virtuous, he said. I was being selfish. He was right. "Try to please." "Think of others first."

These were the lessons I had been taught since my childhood. But I *had* to think of myself first. More than my desire to be loved and accepted, I was afraid of becoming pregnant. Above all, I was terrified of committing a mortal sin. I knew the law of the Church. If I had sex out of wedlock, I would lose my immortal soul for all eternity. I didn't want to hear his arguments. And I didn't want to be thought of as selfish. Finally, I told him I wouldn't see him again.

I was barely passing my courses. But I went out with other young men. I went to college weekends at Yale, M.I.T., Cornell. I took the train from Boston to West Point and went to football games and dances afterwards. One weekend there, while dancing with a senior cadet, I felt extremely hot and faint. He wondered what the red spots were that covered my bare arms and shoulders. I had the German measles. I took the train the next morning from West Point home to Fairfield, where I spent two weeks in bed. As soon as I got back to school in Boston, I spent the next weekend at the Winter Carnival weekend at Middlebury College in Vermont. The more attractive I was to men, the more confident I was that I was someone interesting, charming, sophisticated, smart . . . anyone that another person could love. I absolutely depended on their approval. I craved it. But I never let them touch me. I would rather have been thought unattainable than selfish.

By the end of the winter semester, my grades were dismal. My parents called me, confused and angry. I had no interest in my classes, and I could barely remember why I'd wanted to major in theatre arts at all. I'd never lived away from home, and except for going to classes, this was the first time that I was responsible for myself, for keeping my own hours and running my own life. But in this new, free world that I had yearned for, I was really childlike, self-centered, self-absorbed, confused by my liberty. I didn't want to argue with young men about their desires for sex. Such arguments were too emotional and disturbing. As much as I craved approval and attention, I didn't want to risk being touched. I was frightened. Confused. Tired.

I couldn't think of anything else to do but go to the small, safe society of Fairfield and the security of other people telling me what to do. I wanted to return to the comfort of being controlled. I wanted to go home. I told my parents that I'd given up the idea of being an actress and having a career in the theatre. Why couldn't I just go to a small college near home? I'd major in English, I said. I'd always loved to read. Also, think of the financial savings. Why spend all that money for room and board when I could live at home? My parents didn't argue with me. They agreed. I went home.

CHAPTER TWELVE

Pregnant

I entered Albertus Magnus College, a small Catholic college for young women in a wealthy suburb of New Haven, Connecticut, run by the Dominican nuns. The campus was only an hour away from home on the train, two stops further than Lauralton Hall. The school buildings were converted old mansions that lined Prospect Street, a broad, tree-lined street on the crest of a hill overlooking the city. I decided to major in English and I chose classes in British poetry, modern American literature, mythology, Shakespeare. The Dominicans were a seven-hundred-year-old order of nuns and priests founded by Saint Dominic, a Spanish friar and scholar, to suppress heresy through education. Now, in 1958, the Dominicans were gifted teachers, more interested in education than heresy. Even though we were forbidden to "read, own, sell or otherwise transmit" any book on the "Index of Forbidden Books" under pain of mortal sin, the

Dominicans were liberal and provocative teachers, and to my surprise, I loved my courses. I lost myself in them.

Short, round Sister Mary Patrick gave us her own vivid description of Lord and Lady Macbeth.

"She was young! Much younger than he! She was beautiful! With fiery red hair! Imagine what she thought when she saw him come riding up! Power! She wanted power! She took one look at him and thought, I can have this man's power!"

And the little nun stormed back and forth across the front of the classroom, hands clasped behind her back, head bent forward, turning quickly this way and that, her habit swirling around her and began to quote, first Lady Macbeth, "But screw your courage to the sticking place and we'll not fail!"

Then Sister Mary Patrick turned and faced our class.

"But remember girls, her courage was a fantasy, dependent on others. She had not strength of her own. She came to a sad end. Try not to let that happen to yourselves." And then she quoted from Macbeth.

> Can'st thou not minister to a mind diseased,
> Pluck from the memory a rooted sorrow,
> Raze out the written troubles of the brain,
> And with some sweet oblivious antidote
> Cleanse the bosom of that perilous stuff which weighs upon the heart?
> And the physician answers him:
> Therein the patient must minister to himself.

Life in Fairfield fell back into the familiar routine. College with the nuns on the weekdays, confession on Saturday afternoon, Mass on Sunday. I loved the familiar rituals, the ancient Latin prayers and responses of the Mass. The old hymns that I had learned as a child were the same ones my mother had sung as a girl and that my grandmother had played on the organ when she was young. They were comforting, safe.

Fairfield remained a beautifully preserved colonial town, resistant to change. The town was, in many ways, a symbol of the times. In those days, in the late 1950s, spontaneity frightened people. Emotions were untidy, troublesome, inconvenient. You never disagreed openly with anyone. Such expressions of personal sentiment were in bad taste. You never said exactly what you thought. As my mother always said, "If you can't say anything nice about someone, don't say anything at all." In those days, you went along, you "fit in" with everyone else.

My brother was gone from home. He had joined the Air Force just after he graduated from high school and was stationed in England. I rode my bike alone now along the beach road and toward Penfield Reef. My brother and I had never walked out to the lighthouse. It was too far. How could we have thought we could beat the tide?

I was sad in those days and very lonely. I remembered Macbeth's words, repeated them over and over to myself: "Therein the patient must minister to herself." In an effort to ease my sorrow, which I couldn't understand, and to overcome the loneliness I felt every day, I took my schoolbooks to the library and lost myself in the novels of the Brontë sisters and the poems of Emily Dickinson and Christina Rossetti. I read "In an Artist's Studio" and "The Convent Threshold."

I wept for memory;
She sang for hope that is so fair:
My tears were swallowed by the sea;
Her songs died on the air.

One late afternoon toward the end of the summer of 1959, just before I started my sophomore year at Albertus Magnus, I came home from my summer job in the mail room. My mother told me to go down to the beach and tell my younger sister to come home for dinner. I changed into shorts and T-shirt, took Pepper and went down to the path to the beach. My dog was older and moved more slowly now, but she still loved to swim.

My sister was thirteen that summer, tall and long-legged like our brother and me. She had straight black hair, dark blue eyes and a bridge of freckles across her nose. She was a strong swimmer, and she was taking her last lesson in junior lifesaving. She stood at the water's edge, smiling and talking with the young lifeguard who taught the course. He was tanned, with a sturdy, muscular build and sandy-colored hair. He stood talking to my sister, his arms folded in front of him with the easy physical grace of an athlete used to being watched. My sister pretended not to see Pepper and me as we came down the beach toward them. I thought it was because she wished to avoid dinner, which in our house had become a half-hour of silent eating. My father disliked discussion at the dinner table.

I stood awkwardly for a minute or so before my sister introduced me to the lifeguard. She was possessive of her friends and acquaintances. I suspected that she was having a lonely and sometimes frightening time at home; my father hadn't finished spending his rages. My sister didn't have anyone to take her side, to be a child with, as I'd had. My sister had become distrustful and self-protective. She'd developed a stormy temperament but I understood her perfectly.

Harry was shy and soft-spoken, and he had clear, green eyes and a gentle smile. While Pepper took her swim, we talked for just a few minutes about college, about where I went, and about Fairfield University, the Jesuit University in town, where he was going into his senior year. My sister stood by, her dark eyebrows knit together, fidgeting, jabbing at the sand with her toe.

"Come on," she said to me. "I thought you said dinner was ready. Let's get it over with."

"Okay," I said. I turned to Harry. "It was nice meeting you," I said. I called Pepper and turned to go.

"What are you doing Saturday night?" he said to me. "Some of us from school are going bowling."

"Oh," I said, surprised. "Thank you, but school is starting this week. I'm going to stay home this weekend."

I didn't want to go out. I wanted to be alone. I didn't want any more dates with eager young men. I had been looking forward all summer to returning to school, new class work and weekends of reading at the library . . . solitude.

"Can I call you for some other time?" he said.

"Thanks, but no," I said.

"Well, maybe I'll see you around then," he said.

"Okay," I said. "Bye."

Several weeks later, he did call me to ask me to go to the movies with him. I accepted. I knew why. I was lonely and tired. He picked me up in a new red-and-white Ford convertible, and we drove to the center of town to the same theatre where I'd seen so many movies as a young girl. Afterward we went to Larry's Diner for coffee.

Harry had grown up in Fairfield and graduated from the local high school, where he had been a star basketball player. Though he had offers of basketball scholarships to colleges and universities across the country, he refused them all and chose the local Jesuit University. He was a senior there, majoring in education. He wanted to be a high-school teacher and a basketball coach because, he explained, his own high school years had been the happiest of his life so far and, in a way, he didn't want them to end.

Harry was an only child. His mother, a quiet, timid woman, was single, uneducated and unable to care for him when he was born and so had placed him in foster care when he was an infant. Harry was vague about whether his parents had been married, but he did remember his father, a big, burly man with a shock of sandy-colored hair and a hearty laugh who would alight from a train at the Bridgeport railroad station once every few months, hand him a twenty-dollar bill, pat him on the head, then turn and walk quickly across the tracks to take the next train back to New York.

Harry had no family of his own except his mother. He'd been alone, an outsider in foster families, for all of his childhood. He had no brothers or sisters. He'd never known his grandparents, or even of them. He'd never had a bicycle or a Christmas tree. He did have a single thing from his childhood, a picture of himself as a child of six, a tanned, tow-headed little boy in a neatly pressed white, short-sleeved shirt, kneeling beside a small collie puppy that belonged to the foster family he was staying with. In the picture his face is bent over the puppy, gazing at it, and one arm is bent awkwardly around it as if he is afraid to touch it.

When Harry was eight, his mother married a rough, hard-drinking man some years older than she, the caretaker of a large estate at the top of Greenfield Hill. As the man's drinking increased, he threatened her, and then he beat her. As a boy, Harry saw the beatings. As a teen-ager, he came between his drunken stepfather and terrified mother and took many of the blows intended for her.

When he was sure his mother was safe, Harry escaped the violent atmosphere of his house by losing himself in sports, first in grammar school and then as an all-star high school basketball player, one of the best in New England. His teammates and the coaches took the place of the family he didn't have, and the sport gave him approval and recognition. Colleges from across the country offered him scholarships. He briefly considered one from the Air Force Academy in Colorado, but he turned it down. The Jesuits had offered him a full scholarship to Fairfield University and the new car. He accepted. He would not leave his mother unprotected.

When I met him, Harry had become a devout Catholic. He saw God as his protector, and he was grateful. He was deeply committed to following the rules of the church. They gave him the comfort and security he'd never had. He wanted to meet a nice, young, Catholic woman, settle down and have a big, peaceful family, the kind he'd seen but never had. He wanted a family of his own. He wanted a normal, happy life with a wife who loved him and children. He wanted children, he said.

I wanted to have a family, too, a normal one of my own. I wanted a big, bright house filled with happy, noisy children. I wanted many children, too. I wanted to sit around the dinner table with my husband and children and talk. I wanted a good and gentle husband who would love me and our children. I wanted someone to live for. I thought Harry did, too.

Harry pursued me quietly but persistently. He called me often and then every night. I spent more and more time with him, at first out with his friends from the university and then out with him alone. I went to his basketball games. On Saturday afternoons I sat in the grass on the edge of the softball field and watched him play. Soon we went out together every night on the weekends—to the movies, to parties where he held me close to him as we danced to Johnny Mathis singing "Chances Are" on the phonograph. Harry was a quiet, gentle person, more outwardly restrained than I, but as we spent more and more time together, he grew even more passionate when we kissed. But still I refused to give in to the growing sexual attraction I felt for him. I was afraid of it.

The year was 1959. It wasn't until several years later that the new pope, John XXIII, began to institute the reforms that would free many Catholics from the constraints of the past. At school, the Dominicans were confused at first by the new edicts coming from the Vatican. Soon though, the nuns embraced the changes with their usual intellectual fervor.

But the rules that governed the sexual behavior of Catholics never changed. The primary purpose of sexual intercourse was to create

Catholic children. For the young unmarried Catholic man and woman, the rule was simple, direct, immutable, inviolable. Sexual intercourse outside of marriage was absolutely forbidden—a mortal sin.

As Harry and I spent more time together, we found ourselves depending on each other to ease the loneliness we had endured in the past. When he shared his hopes with me for a happier, more peaceful future, and when he talked about the children he wanted to have, I began to believe that he wanted to marry me. I understood his loneliness. I thought he understood mine. One Sunday afternoon when Harry's mother and stepfather were out, we sat close together on their living room sofa. He put his arms around me and pulled me to him.

"I think I love you," he said. "Do you love me?"

"Yes," I whispered. I did. I loved his quiet, gentle nature. I loved his passion when he kissed me and held me close to him. It made me feel sure he loved me. I needed to feel loved. I needed him to love me. So I didn't stop him when he began to unbutton my blouse. I didn't stop him when he unhooked my bra and held my breasts in his hands. I didn't stop him when he bent and kissed them. I got up and stepped out of my skirt and my underwear. Then I lay down on the sofa and pulled him close to me, on top of me. I had wondered what it would feel like to have a man inside of me. Now I felt a sharp twinge of pain. This was not the erotic experience of the afternoons I'd spent with the senior at Harvard. This was a different sensation, raw, startling, shocking even. Harry got up quickly afterwards as if he were embarrassed, as if I'd caused him to lose control of himself, as if something private in him had been exposed. I felt not embarrassed but ashamed. Awkward. One month later, I was pregnant with my first child. I was nineteen years old.

At first I could not comprehend what had happened to me. My mother was horrified. My father wouldn't even look at me. My parents told no one. I was an object of shame and sin. What would people think of them? Of course I had to marry Harry. I could never even have imagined having an abortion. My parents didn't suggest that I go away, have my baby and give the child up for adoption. I loved Harry, and I didn't want my shame to follow our baby. I had to marry him as soon as possible. I had no choice at all. Neither did Harry. I never even thought that this might be something he didn't want to do. I knew he loved me. He'd said so.

My mother called the pastor, Monsignor Casey, and made an appointment for me to see him. She drove me to the rectory at four o'clock on a rainy afternoon in late April and dropped me off. I was two months pregnant. As I walked up the flagstone path to the big double front doors to the rectory there was the faint, sweet smell of forsythia from the gardens in back. The fragrance made me nauseous. I rang the bell and the housekeeper answered. She showed me into a small, dark room to the left of the hallway, and I sat down on a stiff leather sofa to wait for the Monsignor. I waited for a half hour. I heard the rustle of his cassock in the hallway and I stood up, expecting him to come into the room. He did not. He stayed in the hall.

"What is it you want?" he said.

"I need your permission to marry, Father," I said.

"You don't have it," he said. "You will not marry in this parish. Make some other arrangement." And he turned to go.

"What?" I said. "Why?"

"You know very well why. Your parents told me that you are pregnant. You have disgraced yourself and your family. What would the rest of this parish think if I allowed you to be married in this church? You will not disgrace this parish." He turned and left.

I felt my cheeks flush, and I began to tremble. I sat down on the leather sofa. I heard the rustle of a cassock again in the hall. I stood up again. The new curate came into the room and shut the door. He was young, in his late twenties, burly and broad-shouldered, with pale, almost delicate features. He had a small, straight nose, fine brown hair and soft blue eyes. I'd seen him after Mass on several Sundays.

"Are you all right, Susan?" he said quietly. I wondered how he knew my name.

"Yes," I said. "May I call my mother? She said she would pick me up outside the church."

"Call her and tell her to pick you up here. You look pale."

"Thank you, Father, but she said she wouldn't come to the rectory."

"Why not?"

"I don't know, Father. She wouldn't say."

"Well, call her then, and you and I will go over to the church. Tell her we'll meet her there."

"Excuse me, Father, but I don't think she wants you to see her."

"Oh," he said, and sighed. "That's too bad. The problem is yours, not your mother's."

We walked over to the church and went in through one of the side doors. We sat down in one of the pews. The church was empty and silent. There was the familiar scent of candle wax and incense. The statues of Saint Thomas the Apostle and Saint Agnes stood in their niches, racks of white votive lights flickering in front of them. High above the altar was the same faded painting of the Ascension of Christ, his eyes raised to heaven as if disgusted with everything on earth. In the shadows of the sanctuary, near to the altar, stood the tall, white statue of the Madonna with her outstretched hands and inscrutable face. There were the deep red velvet curtains of the confessionals, on each side of the church. I began to shiver in my raincoat. He took my hand.

"Should I make a confession?" I said.

"Are you sorry?" he whispered.

"Yes."

"For what, Susan?"

"I'm sorry for everything." Tears filled my eyes and ran down my cheeks. "I'm sorry for all my sins."

"God knows," said the young priest. He put his arm around me.

"I don't know what to do, Father."

"Don't cry, now," he said. "I'll take care of you."

We walked out of the church into the early evening darkness. I had no idea how long we had sat there, together in the pew. I had no idea what would happen to me next. I did know that I trusted the young priest. I saw my mother's car parked in the shadows of the parking lot next to the church.

"Thank you, Father," I said.

"Don't worry," he said and pressed my hand. Then he turned and walked toward the rectory.

࿇࿇࿇࿇࿇

The young priest arranged for Harry and I to be married two days later on a Thursday morning in a church fifty miles away, in Hartford. The short, early morning ceremony would be performed by one of his friends from the seminary who had been ordained with him. The ceremony would take place at 7:45 A.M., between the regular daily masses. We had to be on time.

The church was over an hour away. My father drove. My mother sat next to him. They stared straight ahead without speaking. I sat in the back seat. We picked Harry up at his mother's house at 6:30 A.M. It was a dark, rainy morning. Harry wore a tan raincoat over his suit and tie. I wore a gray tweed suit. The skirt was too tight around my thickening waist, and the buttons of the jacket strained across my swelling breasts.

Harry got into the car and sat silently on the far side of the back seat next to the window. I moved over closer to him and reached for his hand and took it. He turned to look at me with a brief, tight smile. "I love you," I whispered. He said nothing. He looked down at my hand and patted it. Then he withdrew it and pulled the collar of his raincoat up close around his neck. He turned and stared out the window.

No organ rumbled and burst forth into majestic strains of Lohengrin on our wedding day. I didn't come down the aisle in a long, white bridal dress on my father's arm to meet my new husband at the altar. The church wasn't filled with happy relatives to wish us joy. There was no mass. There were no flowers. No bridesmaids. No friends. And it was all my own fault.

Our witnesses were the church janitor and his wife, the house-keeper of the rectory. He wore a dark blue maintenance uniform. She wore a gray housedress. My mother and father stood as close as they could to the altar and watched as Harry and I repeated our vows after the priest. It was the only time Harry spoke.

On the way back to Fairfield, we stopped at a Howard Johnson's for our wedding breakfast. Harry and I sat together in a booth facing my parents. My parents were silent. I tried to engage them in polite small talk for Harry's sake.

"Wasn't the priest nice?" I said.

"He was in a hurry," my mother said.

"Well, he had to say a mass right after us," I said.

My mother said nothing.

"I forgot that we had to have witnesses," I said. "It was nice of those two people to stand up for us."

My father stared at me. "Some people are responsible," he said.

I knew he was right. Some people were responsible. I was not one of them. My father and mother had been responsible for me and my sister and my brothers. They had sheltered us, fed us, clothed us. They had made sure that our teeth were straightened, that we went to the best schools they could afford and they had sacrificed many things they would have liked so they could care for us first. How had I repaid them for their sacrifices and kindnesses? I'd done nothing for them but think of myself.

I put my arm through Harry's.

"Everything will be fine, Dad," I said. "We're going to make a good life together. You'll be proud of us."

I smiled at Harry next to me. He turned to look at me. He smiled a brief, sad smile. I saw that he was trapped.

My parents didn't want us to live together because they didn't want anyone to know we were married. When Harry graduated in several months and it became obvious that I was pregnant, they planned to announce our marriage. After that we could find an apartment of our own and begin our life together. We dropped Harry off at his mother's house. I went to my parents' house with them.

I changed from my tweed suit to a loose-fitting dress and walked down to the Post Road to take the bus into Bridgeport to the Butler Business School where I'd enrolled to learn how to type. I needed to find a job, anything that would help Harry to support our new family and I had to work for as long as I could. I'd had to drop out of Albertus Magnus. What kind of example was I to my classmates? Couldn't I have waited to marry and have children until I graduated, like all the other young women? How could I have gone to school pregnant, in maternity clothes? In those days it was out of the question. The nuns would not allow it.

Butler Business School was on the second floor of a run-down brick building that had been an old printing factory. I climbed the stairs to a long, high-ceilinged classroom where rows of women sat in front of cumbersome, black typewriters. At the sound of a small bell, they turned their heads smartly to the right and looked down at the notepads of dictation on their desks, hands poised in the air over their typewriters like the claws of thin, anxious birds. Then they began to type in unison, their fingers flashing and leaping along the keys. The clacking noise of the typewriters was deafening. It made me dizzy and nauseous. I went into the ladies room and sat down alone on a metal chair and fought the nausea until it passed. I was nineteen years old. My husband was twenty-one. I was afraid that he might not love me. I had brought shame on everyone. And it was all my own fault.

෴෴෴

L ooking back, I wondered. Why had I done it? For approval? For the need to be loved? I was so lonely, in those days, without myself.

CHAPTER THIRTEEN

Therein the Patient Must Minister to Herself: Day Five

I called Annie first thing in the morning. "Annie, I want to tell you to speak up about what's important to you, okay?"

"Mom! What are you talking about?"

"Well, yesterday when you were here you kept your worries to yourself and entertained everybody first."

"So? I didn't want anybody to know I was worried. I wanted everybody to just be happy and not think about sickness or anything."

"It's okay to share your worries."

"I know, but I feel better when I make people laugh."

"It's not your job to make other people happy."

There was silence on the other end of the phone. "Annie?"

"Why are you telling me this stuff?"

"I've been doing lots of thinking and reading since I've been here. When I was young I always wanted approval from everybody. I didn't have any inside strength of my own. Now I'm trying to find it.

Promise me you'll be yourself and not worry about what other people are thinking."

"Okay, Mom." But she did want approval. A lesson learned from me. I had tried to give my children strength, but had I passed on my weaknesses instead? How could I help her? Was it too late for me to teach her, for her to learn? I picked up the Evans book from my nightstand and began to read. "The individual . . . is strong and self-reliant; the collective person is . . . trying to accommodate himself to all. Development of individuality is a safeguard to life and health. It lifts a person out of the collective authority. The process of lifting one's self above its influence is indeed difficult. It requires such strength of character as does not grow overnight." That was the answer. I would have to become stronger, self-reliant. Then I could show Annie by example.

A short time later Dr. McCullough came in with Rita. He looked at the Evans book in my lap. "What are you reading?" he said.

"*A Psychological Study of Cancer,*" I said.

"Hmmm," he said. "I thought it would be one of your books for school."

"No," I said. "I can always read those. I seem to be like the cancer patients she's writing about."

"What does she say about them?"

"She thinks they're people who live outside of themselves, for others. They don't live for themselves. And when they lose the thing they've been living for, that's when trouble comes."

"Haven't you been living for yourself?"

"No."

"Why not?"

"I don't know," I said. "I always believed that would be selfish . . . to live for myself. The truth is, I guess I never thought I was that important."

"Really?" He looked surprised and then confused. He stared at me now, even longer. "Well, you are."

"I am what?"

"Important."

"Thank you," I said. I felt embarrassed.

"I want to take a look at that bandage," he said.

Rita came in to help him. He took off the gauze that covered the right side of my chest. I forced myself to look down at the place where my breast had been. I saw that a long, raw scar ran down my chest, all the way from my shoulder to the top of my rib cage. Instinctively, I put both hands up to cover the empty place. Oh, my poor breast! Where had it gone? I would never see it again, ever, never, anymore. I felt tears slip down my cheeks. I could feel my shoulders heaving but I wasn't crying. The doctor wrapped another bandage around my chest and then he took my hand. He stood holding it silently. After several moments, I felt I could speak. "I'm all right," I said. "Thank you."

"We had to go back and take care of that hemorrhage," he said. "That's why the scar looks so bad right now. It will heal."

I felt the tears sliding down my face again.

"What did you do with it?" I whispered.

"With what?" he said. "What did I do with what?"

"My breast."

I saw him glance at the nurse.

"We took care of it," he said.

Andrew came with Harry later that afternoon. He was fifteen then, a tall, blond, blue-eyed boy who looked like his father but had inherited my emotional nature. He was bright and sensitive, but impetuous and sometimes reckless. His emotions often ruled him.

"Ma!" He put his arms around me and hugged me carefully. "Ma! Are you okay? You look great! Where is your bandage? Oh! It doesn't look like anything is missing! You're fine, right? When will you get out?"

"Soon!" I said.

Andrew rushed headlong into everything when he was a little boy. He wanted to dive off the highest diving boards or ride his bike the fastest down the steepest hills. I worried about his safety, but Harry reminded me that he had to learn some caution on his own; he had to learn to be careful about himself. At fifteen, Andrew was more cautious and, since the divorce, pensive and anxious. And then he had received the frightening phone call from the nurse.

"He just wanted to make sure you were okay for himself," said Harry.

"I'm fine," I said. "I just want to get out of here."

Before they left, Andrew leaned over to kiss me good-bye.

"That nurse scared me," he said. "But you don't look sick at all."

"I had a hemorrhage," I said. "But I'm cured. I'm in control. Don't be frightened anymore."

"Okay," he said. "I'll see you next week! For Thanksgiving vacation! I love you, Ma."

"I love you, too, Andrew."

Harry leaned down and kissed my cheek. "Are you sure you're alright?" he said.

"Pretty sure," I whispered. "I'll call you."

Andrew was still in the doorway. He looked frightened. I saw there were tears in his eyes.

"Andrew!" I said. "I love you. There's no reason to be afraid."

"Okay, Ma." He smiled one of the sad, sweet smiles so like his father's. What was he thinking? Was he afraid of losing me again? He turned and left with Harry.

Did my children know I had cancer? I had vowed not even to say the word to them. I wanted to wait, to be sure I was well. Then I could tell them it was something I'd had but didn't have anymore.

My children's lives had spun out of their control because of me. What other fears and grief could I bring them? I felt the old, too-familiar pangs of guilt rise up in me and tears stung my eyes.

Dana, now eighteen, was a gentle, quiet girl with a shy smile. Since the divorce she had become unsure of herself, and like Annie, too anxious to please. Had she, too, been studying me for all these years? She joined the Air Force right after she graduated from high school and she'd never returned to Connecticut. It was almost as if she couldn't get far enough away from home. I thought of my brother. Had my daughter done the same thing he had years before and escaped from chaos to the order and security of the Air Force?

Annie was, like Andrew, fearful and anxious. The divorce was an event that had happened to them, and it was out of their control. Was Annie's charming bravado her way of controlling a world that I'd sent spinning when I divorced her father? Would Andrew be able to control his anxiety?

Peggy was a freshman at the University of Connecticut. I'd been in the hospital for days now, and I still hadn't heard from her. I'd seen her last in September, just before she left for college. Then she seemed preoccupied, distant. She wanted to become an actress and I'd done for her what I'd promised. The day after she graduated, she came into New York and met every agent I knew. They were enchanted with her and sent her out on auditions immediately. She'd already made a television commercial and was making the long commute from college in Storrs, Connecticut, into New York for more auditions. Was she too busy? Was this why I hadn't heard from her? Or was it because of Pat? She'd met him once during the summer. I watched her eyes flicker over his face, taking in every part of it, his dark eyes and his full mouth. She was aloof to him, cool, as if she wanted him to believe she didn't like him. Did she think he would take me away from her? Was she protecting herself from further hurt? I didn't know.

I had cost my children the security I had tried to give them and the strength I had encouraged them to find. Now they were anxious, fearful, self-protective and self-absorbed. I'd failed them as a mother. Would they ever forgive me? *I'll never know*, I thought. *I have no more strength to keep on going. It's easier to give up.* The woman in the bed next to me had visitors. I hid my face in my hands to hide my tears.

I felt a comforting hand on my foot. Dr. Siegel was standing next to my bed. He handed me a box of tissues from the nightstand. I dried my eyes.

"Remember what I told you last time? That it's okay to love yourself?"

"I can't concentrate on myself. I just think I've made so many mistakes. It seems to me that when I did think of myself I disappointed so many people! I caused such grief for everyone! I keep thinking about all of them!" I had started to cry again. I was mortified. He handed me one of the tissues.

"Who's perfect?" he asked. "Did you ever think that maybe we're all perfectly imperfect? Why don't you try forgiving yourself? That's a start. Forgive yourself. That way you'll start to care for yourself."

"I've been trying to understand myself," I said. "I think I know what happened. I spent most of my life so far trying to please other people. I was living for other people. I was my mother's daughter, my children's mother, my husband's wife. I lost myself somewhere along the line. Now it's hard to figure out how to live for me, to forgive myself. Sometimes I wonder if there's a 'me' there."

"Oh yes, there is," he said. "You'll find yourself when you learn how to forgive yourself. Then you'll be amazed at the way you'll love everyone else. You know, you can give to others without giving yourself away."

"I guess I don't know how to do that yet," I said.

"You'll learn," he said. "I have faith in you!" He smiled his broad, happy grin. "Do your visualizations! I told you they can be powerful. That's one way to start caring for you."

"Thank you, Doctor."

"Bernie. I told you! Bernie!"

"Thank you, Bernie." He grinned again and went to the door. There he stopped and turned around. "Another thing. Illness isn't your failure. It can be the way you change your life."

I found myself remembering Sister Mary Pat striding back and forth in front of our classroom at Albertus Magnus. The little Dominican nun understood the tragedy of Lady Macbeth. "Remember girls, she had not strength of her own. She came to a sad end. Try not to let that happen to yourselves." I remembered again the lines from Macbeth. "Can'st thou not pluck from memory a rooted sorrow . . . and cleanse the bosom of that perilous stuff which weighs upon the brain?" And the physician answers: "Therein the patient must minister to herself."

I closed my eyes and imagined the most powerful cells in my body fighting those that were diseased. I imagined my own immune system ministering to me. I imagined . . . and then let my body do its healing.

Just before sleep I picked up Elida Evans's book again and tried to read. But I couldn't get Andrew's tear-stained face out of my mind. I saw again his sweet sad, smile and I thought again of Harry . . . and the family I had had.

I looked over at the woman in the bed next to me. Her visitors had left. She lay still, as quiet and removed as always. Her family came dutifully every night, but she barely acknowledged them. They stayed for a half-hour, sitting silently around her bed, and then one would catch the eyes of another and glance toward the door. They stood up and filed past the woman, each one placing a kiss on her forehead before leaving the room.

Now her husband remained, as he did every night, sitting at the side of her bed, silent, resigned, remote, fingering his rosary beads, his lips moving soundlessly in prayer. "What's the use of that?" I wondered to myself. "Why doesn't he talk to her instead?" I thought of Harry on our wedding day. Our marriage had been full of silences. If only we could have known. . . .

തന്റെതന്റെ

I gave birth to my first baby on a snowy morning in early December 1960. A nurse placed her, a warm, tight little bundle, in my arms. She had long black hair that curled at her neck and black eyelashes that lay softly against the perfect curve of her cheek. Her mouth was like a tiny rosebud that, as I looked down at her, opened unexpectedly in an exquisite yawn. My parents were delighted with my baby daughter. My mother was thrilled with her. She sat in my hospital room and cradled her and sang to her. Gifts and flowers arrived from my aunts and friends of my parents. The shame of my pregnancy had vanished.

Harry drove us home to our new apartment through streets that were still snow-covered. Our new apartment was on the top floor of a three-family house on a quiet residential street in Fairfield, about five miles from my parents' house. He helped me carefully up the three flights of stairs and then left to return to Fairfield Prep, where he'd gotten a job as a math teacher and basketball coach. He worked long hours, teaching all day then staying after school for basketball practice into the evening.

My mother came with a casserole she had made for our dinner and stayed to show me how to diaper the baby and make her formula and pour it into the sterilized glass bottles with rubber nipples. Then she went home.

That night I laid my baby in a bassinette next to my bed, but I dared not close my eyes. Who would watch her? What if I didn't hear her cries when she woke in the night? What if I hadn't prepared the formula properly? What if she got sick? We lived on the third floor. What if there was a fire? Finally I drifted to sleep. When her cries woke me later I saw that Harry was asleep on the other side of the bed. I got up and changed the baby's diaper and came back to Harry's side of the bed. He was awake, staring at me.

"Would you hold her for a minute while I get her bottle?" I said.

"I can't," he said.

"What?"

"No. I've never held a baby. I don't know how. No."

"Just sit up," I said. "I'll put her in your arms. All you have to do is hold her."

"No," he said. He got up, went out to the living room and laid down on the sofa. "I have to sleep," he said. "I have to teach in the morning."

"Of course," I said. "You're right."

I laid the baby down in the bassinette and went out to the kitchen to warm her bottle. She began to wail pitifully. I picked her up again, took her with me into the kitchen and rocked her while I warmed her bottle. Then I took her back into the bedroom, shut the door and sat down on the bed to feed her.

I sat for hours holding her. How could she be so small, yet so full of life? Her tiny fingers had beautiful almond-shaped fingernails. Her perfect pink toes curled when I kissed them. I lifted her so that her head lay on my shoulder and rested my cheek against the fine softness of her dark hair. I adored her. Two months later, on the day my first baby, Dana, was Christened, I knew I was pregnant with my second. I was disbelieving at first. I would have two babies not even a year apart.

Harry and I were both devout Catholics. The Catholic couple was forbidden to use contraceptives, and the Catholic wife was forbidden to refuse her husband's request for sex. But Harry had told me before we were married that he wanted children. I hoped he would be happy.

But he made no comment when I told him I was pregnant with our second child. Instead he looked at me with a pained expression, as if the new baby I was carrying would be too great a burden for him. I was shocked.

"But I thought you wanted lots of kids!"

"I didn't think you'd have another this soon. It's okay, I'll just have to get an extra job," he said. "I'm sure we can stay in this apartment, at least for another year."

He began to spend more and more time at school. He was studying for his master of math degree, and to earn extra money, he now coached baseball and basketball in addition to teaching. Saturday mornings he went to the university library to study. Saturday afternoons and Sunday mornings he played basketball or softball at the Fairfield Boys club. He was rarely at home. When he was, on some Sunday afternoons, he lost himself in football or basketball or baseball games on television. Most Friday nights he played poker with his old friends from high school. One Friday night in the spring, when our daughter was several months old and slept through the night, I suggested we get a baby-sitter and go out to the movies.

"I don't see you very often," I said. "I miss you."

"I'm working very hard to support you and the baby," he said. "And now we have another one on the way."

"I know," I said. "But couldn't we spend more time together?"

"What do you want," he said simply. "All my time?"

"No!" I said. "I just thought you'd like to be home more."

"I'll have the guys over here for poker then," he said.

"I meant just the two of us," I said.

"I don't like to argue," he said. "If you don't want the guys over here, just say so."

I felt embarrassed and selfish. I said no more.

I filled my days taking the baby for long walks around the neighborhood in her carriage. Some afternoons my mother picked me up, and we did the grocery shopping. She gave me her old sewing machine and I learned to sew. I spent evenings making curtains and slipcovers for our apartment.

My grandmother still came up from New York to spend an occasional weekend with my mother and father. One of my aunts would bring her, or my mother would drive into the city to pick her up. She was in her early eighties now and increasingly frail. I spent hours with her at my mother's house, learning to make little dresses for my daughter. She brought me fine, pale pink and white cotton lawn and taught me how to shirr and hand-smock the dresses. Once, as I sat with her cutting fabric and patterns, I saw her studying my face with a certain look of sadness.

"What is it, Gram?" I said.

"Are you happy, dear girl?"

"Yes!" I said. "Of course! I married a good man. He never had a family of his own. He works very hard to support me and the baby."

"I didn't ask about him or your baby," she said. "I asked about you."

"What did you ask me?"

She looked at me for a long moment.

"Let's take a turn, dear."

We went out of the house and walked down to the beach. She put her arm in mine as we walked. We walked slowly along the beach path and then stopped and stood together at the top of the beach. She was frail now, but she held her head high. She looked far out over the water. She turned to me. Her eyes were the color of the pale, blue sky.

"I asked you if you were happy," she said.

I couldn't answer her.

"It's always mind over matter, Susan."

"What do you mean?"

"I mean that we are able to think ourselves above our problems.

The mind is powerful. Trust it. Make your own happiness, Susan. You must take care of yourself."

My Grandmother Ryan died several months later. She had been my greatest friend.

At the end of that summer, a friend from my days at Boston University called me. She wanted me to visit her and her family at their summer house on Cape Cod for two weeks with my little girl. I couldn't wait to go. Harry was rarely at home, and I was lonely. I was tired, too, from months of quiet worry about the emptiness of my marriage. Before we were married Harry had been affectionate, even passionate. But in the year since we had been married, he was distant and detached. He rarely talked to me, never touched me and avoided me when I tried to kiss him. On the rare occasions when we had sex he turned away from me and fell quickly asleep. He was embarrassed if I asked him if he had enjoyed our sex together. And he was embarrassed by the way I looked as I went further along in my second pregnancy. Several times I saw him looking sadly at my full, round stomach as if the sight of it reminded him of a mistake he kept making.

I came home from Cape Cod on a Sunday afternoon. Harry met me at the door. He told me that he'd had a young woman there, staying with him while I was gone. He cried when he told me. I stood in the doorway, heavy with our second child, holding our older baby in my arms, surrounded by baby things: a stroller, a fold-up playpen, her brightly colored plastic toys, our suitcases from the trip.

"I had to tell you," he said.

"Why?" I said.

"I was afraid you might hear it from someone else," he said.

He stood, waiting for me to say something. But I couldn't think of anything.

I took the baby into her room and put her down in her crib. When I came back out into the living room, Harry was gone. I went to the living room window and looked down into the street below. I saw him get into his car, pull away from the curb and drive down the street to the corner. The car paused briefly, but then turned the corner and disappeared.

I went about putting everything from our trip away, as if by habit. I fed the baby and gave her a bath. She sat in the tub and slapped her little hands at the water, splashing and chortling. I put her down for her nap. I did the laundry. I went out to the back porch with the basket of clean, wet diapers and hung them in neat, white squares on the clothesline that stretched from our top-floor apartment to the one across the yard. I took the vacuum cleaner out and vacuumed every inch of the apartment. I went back into the bedroom and pulled the bedspread off the bed. The sheets had just been changed and were fresh and clean. The baby had wakened and was cooing and laughing softly to herself in her crib. I went in and picked her up. She had her father's gentle, green eyes. What had happened to him? Why?

What had happened to the laughing, blond young man who came to pick me up in his red and white Ford convertible every Friday night? Who took me to the dances at his school and held me close to him while Johnny Mathis sang "Chances Are" on the phonograph? I did not know. But I had to know. What had happened to his gentle smile? To his hopes, which I thought had been so like mine?

He hadn't known what it meant to be a father or husband. Suddenly, at twenty-one, before he could fulfill any of the dreams he might have had, he was both. What must it have been like for him on the morning of our wedding, sitting across from my parents, trapped with me in that booth in Howard Johnson's? A Catholic marriage was a permanent union. Only death could terminate it.

We'd known each other for only five months before I was pregnant. How could we have realized in that brief time that we should never have married at all? I was emotional and immature. He was restrained and reticent. Now I realized that the only thing we'd had in common was our loneliness. How could we have built a future on that? I thought of his sadness. How could I ease it? What troubled him? I must be to blame. How? What had I done? What had I not done?

I gave the baby her dinner and sat down with her in the living room to wait for Harry to come home. I remembered the rules. The Catholic wife was forbidden to deny her husband's request for sex. I had never denied Harry's rare request for sex. In the Catholic marriage, to have sex meant to have children. He had always said he wanted children. Was that the truth? If only he would tell me. We could abstain from sex until the "safe" time of the month!

Hours went by. I put the baby to bed and went back into the darkened living room to wait. Why did he want sex with another woman and not with me when I was always so willing? Was I too willing? If I'd been a "good" girl and remained a virgin until our wedding night, would he have loved me more? There were so many questions. I couldn't think of a single answer.

I fell asleep in the darkness, sitting in the chair. I woke as Harry came quietly up the stairs and into our apartment. I saw him slip into the bedroom. I got up and went after him. He was sitting on his side of the bed, his back to me.

"Please talk to me," I said. "I can't understand what happened."

"I screwed up," he said. "That's what happened."

I went over to him and eased myself down next to him.

"Have I disappointed you in some way?" I said.

He turned and looked at me for a long moment.

"This was a mistake," he said.

His eyes filled with tears. He put his head down.

"Did I cause it?" I said.

"We both caused it," he said. "It should never have happened."

"What?"

"All of it."

"What can I do?"

"Nothing," he said. "Don't you understand? You can't do anything."

"It's all right," I said. "I love you."

I went to put my arm around him. He pulled away from me.

"Leave me alone," he said. "Please leave me alone."

He got up and went out into the living room. I went after him.

"I love you," I said.

"I know," he said. "Good night."

Our second daughter was born two months later, on a November morning, a week before the Thanksgiving of 1961. She had a mass of dark, curly hair, a perfect, heart-shaped face and pale blue eyes. She lay in my arms and gazed up at me as if wondering how she had arrived.

"Hello, little girl," I said. "You came straight from heaven."

She continued to study me.

"It's true," I told her. "God sent you."

She stared up at me until sleep overtook her, and she slept. I adored her. I named her Margaret Mary Emily, for my mother and my grandmother.

Harry brought us home on Thanksgiving Day. Our apartment was crowded with my aunts, my friend Jessie, who was on her way back into New York from New Haven, my sister and my brother, who was home from England on leave. We sat in the living room, each one taking a turn holding the new baby while I held my older daughter, who was not quite one year old. She had stayed with my mother while I was in the hospital and had missed me, my sister said. Now she wouldn't leave my lap. Later, after everyone had left, I sat holding both of my daughters while I gave the new one her bottle. Harry had gone to bed. I sat there long into the night with my babies.

I felt liberated on that night, there with both of my daughters sleeping in my arms, as if finally I had solved a lingering problem. My duty was to be at home caring for the children. In those days, that was the custom and I intended to follow it. As I looked at my baby daughters, it occurred to me that I was like a bow and they were the arrows. I would do my best to direct them, but I could only hope that once they had left me they would live their lives in such a way as to arrive in heaven. I vowed to encourage them to be themselves. My hopes were for them.

I was a young Catholic wife living in an empty marriage at a time when divorce was out of the question. I would make the very best out of my situation. On that night I knew that my marriage was a partnership to care for the children, and I was determined to give them the security and love of a family that I vowed to make as normal as I could. And somehow I hoped that if I could give Harry that same security and love, we might become closer. I was twenty-two years old.

At first my days and nights were filled caring for two little ones, but after several months my infant daughter began to sleep through the night and our lives resumed a normal pattern. We moved from the third-floor apartment to a larger one in Fairfield on the ground floor. I put the two little girls in their carriage and walked to the grocery store until we bought a second car, an old blue and white Chevy sedan. Then I drove to the Goodwill store and bought used furniture; old dressers and end tables, and a wooden table and chairs for the kitchen. I piled the stuff into the trunk of the old car and brought it home, and while the girls took their afternoon naps, I stripped and refinished the pieces. I bought fabric, and after the girls were asleep at night I made dresses for them and more slipcovers and curtains for the new apartment. I went to bed early and fell asleep alone. Harry earned his masters degree and took on more coaching duties to earn extra money. We were like every other young married couple in those days except that we were never together.

My mother stopped in one afternoon before the little girls took their nap. She was knitting matching green cardigan sweaters for them, and she wanted to fit the sleeves. We sat at the kitchen table while little Peggy crawled busily around on the floor between the table legs. She hauled herself up, clutching my legs, and then toddled back and forth between my mother and me. She lost her balance, sat down suddenly on the floor and then laughed uproariously at herself. Dana brought first one doll, then another for my mother to inspect. I caught my mother staring at me.

"You're too thin," she said.

"I'm always thin," I said.

"Yes, I know. But now you're skinny. You look tired. Why don't you lay down with the girls when they take their nap?"

"Because I can get a lot done while they're sleeping."

"Well, that's what being married is all about. Taking care of other people."

"I know."

"But I'm worried about you," she said. "Is anything wrong?"

"No!" I said. "Mom, you remember when we were little! There's so much to do. It's hectic."

"Well, try to get more rest," she said. "You're sure there's nothing wrong?"

"There's nothing wrong."

I never told her. I never told anyone about the awesome loneliness of my marriage. But I knew I was alone. I remembered my grand-mother's last words to me: "You must make your own happiness." I understood that I had to make an adult life for myself within the boundaries of my marriage—and I resolved to do it.

So, one afternoon a short time later, I picked up the telephone and called the head of the drama department at Fairfield University. The school was renovating an old garage on the campus for use as a small theatre. The opening production was to be *The Glass Menagerie* by Tennessee Williams. Auditions were to be held in several weeks. I decided to go. I told no one. I didn't want anyone to tell me I couldn't . . . or that I shouldn't. I didn't want to hear that I was being foolish or selfish. I might have believed them.

I hired a baby-sitter the night of the auditions and drove to the campus. I pulled into the parking lot outside the theatre and turned off the car. But I didn't go in to the theatre. I sat in my car, outside in the twilight. I saw other people, young men and women my age, going into the theatre. What was I doing, anyway? Who did I think I was? I was Harry's wife. I was a young mother with two little girls. What would people think if I was out every night rehearsing for a play? What would he think? My place was in the home. I started the car, backed out of the parking lot and drove home.

As I pulled up in front of our apartment I saw the baby-sitter inside through the window, sitting by herself in front of the television. In my mind's eye, I saw myself, sitting, head bent over my sewing machine, sewing . . . alone. I realized that my children were safe in their beds and that Harry wasn't home to miss me. "I just can't be alone anymore," I said. "I hope he'll understand. He has to understand!" I pulled away from the apartment and drove back to the theatre.

The Glass Menagerie is a play about a small Southern family, deserted by the husband and trapped by the Depression. The sister, Laura, is a crippled young woman who escapes the harsh reality of their lonely life by losing herself in a world of little glass animals. Her brother, Tom, escapes by going to the movies and "manufacturing illusions." Amanda, their mother, escapes into dreams of her past but longs to secure a bright future for her already grown children. There is a gentleman caller in the play, the only one from the world of reality: "The long delayed but always expected something that we live for." He is Laura's last hope for romance and a normal life.

The lobby of the small theatre was brightly lit and filled with people waiting to audition. There were young men from the university trying out for the part of Tom or the gentleman caller, other young women in their early twenties and several older women there to audition for Amanda. I waited my call to audition, and when it came I walked into the darkened theatre. Inside there was a simple stage lit only by a single spotlight. There were two chairs under the spotlight, side by side. I stepped onto the stage and into the spotlight. A voice came from somewhere in the center of the theatre.

"Would you read with the gentleman caller, Susan?" I looked out into the darkness that was so familiar to me . . . the intimate darkness that I remembered. It had been a magical darkness, full of anticipation and mystery. The director was sitting in the center of one of the middle rows. He was an aesthetic-looking older man with a neatly trimmed goatee and thinning hair. His face looked luminous, disembodied in the spill of light from the stage.

"It's the last part of the last scene," he said. A young man, one of the students came up onto the stage to read with me. "Please begin," said the director. I felt the old excitement flood through me as I began to read: "My glass collection takes up a good deal of my time . . ."

The director's voice almost startled me. "Susan, would you please stay? I'd like to speak to you afterwards."

I won the part of Laura, the crippled girl. No one minded. Harry seemed content that I had found a way to occupy myself. But for me winning the role meant much more. It meant that I was a success at something. This acting . . . the make-believe . . . was something I was good at. People would applaud at the end of my performance. I knew that I would transport and please them. They would approve of me. And I would become someone else, someone who mattered, someone who was "real," if only for a little while.

But I had no other illusions. I couldn't really escape into a world of fantasy like the one Laura found in her glass menagerie. The theatre would never hold the magic for me that it once had. There was no future in it for me. It was not a real world, but it was a world where I'd been happy once and I had my memories.

The play ran for three weeks. At the end I asked the director why he had chosen me for the role.

"Because when I look at you I see Laura," he said. Then he quoted Tennessee Williams: "When you look at a piece of delicately spun glass you think of two things: how beautiful it is and how easily it can be broken."

I didn't realize then that I was as fragile and crippled as the young woman I was playing.

CHAPTER FOURTEEN

Silences

As the years went on, Harry and I achieved a strange kind of peace. We never argued. We treated each other in that polite but distant manner peculiar to unhappily married couples. There were times when I thought we had come closer together. We had two more children, Andrew in 1964 and Annie two years later. When she was born, we had four children under six years of age. In time, I stopped worrying and wondering about Harry's distant manner, and I tried to accept it as part of his character. I had always loved his quiet, gentle nature. I had thought that he was nothing like my father. But had I married a man as removed in his way as my father was in his?

And why had I been so attracted to him, really? Perhaps to understand my father? To understand a man who either wouldn't or couldn't love me? But I never understood Harry. I never understood how he could have changed so completely from the caring young

· man I'd dated to the distant man he became on the very day of our wedding. He was, for all the time I was married to him, an enigma. Even so, in those days I loved him.

We moved away from Fairfield to the hills of western Connecticut. Harry's father gave us the downpayment and we bought a new house on two acres of wooded land, a colonial with four bedrooms and a fireplace in the living room. Harry left his job at Fairfield Prep and taught math at the public high school in our town, doubling his salary. He left for school at six in the morning then stayed to coach a sport into the late afternoon: basketball in winter, baseball in spring.

When Dana was old enough to go to school, I started months in advance to make her school dresses. Peggy begged to go to kindergarten, but we told her she was too young and that she would have to wait until the next year. She was heartbroken. I went to the school principal and asked if she could attend, although in a different class. Because my daughters were so close in age, the principal agreed. Dana went to the morning session, and Peggy went in the afternoon. Early in the morning on the first day of school, Peggy watched from the front door as Dana climbed onto the school bus. Then she went upstairs and dressed herself, hours before the bus would pick her up. She came down to the dining room and dragged a chair over to the window and sat down to wait for her bus, her book bag and lunch box on the floor next to her. She was a happy, carefree little girl, but this day I could see her blonde head bent seriously over one of her storybooks, and I saw how intently she stared up the driveway for the first glimpse of the school bus. As soon as it appeared over the brow of our hill, she called out to me.

"Mom! Mom! It's here!"

We went up the driveway and waited as the bus rolled up. The doors opened and Dana jumped down with some of the other little ones from our neighborhood. They wore little red paper circles with their names printed in bold black letters pinned to their dresses and shirts. Peggy stared at the name tags with round eyes. But at the door to the bus, Peggy hesitated. She turned back to look at me and I saw that her eyes were filled with tears.

"Mom! I can't go!" she cried.

"Why, Peg?"

"I can't get on! I can't go to school if I'm too little!"

I saw that her little legs were too short to make the first step up into the bus. "Of course you can go," I said. I lifted her and watched as she took her seat next to the window. She waved to me, her tears gone and a look of pure joy on her face. I met the school bus every day that year to lift her on and then catch her as she jumped off, her arms stretched out to me and blonde hair flying, until she could climb up and down the steps to the school bus herself.

While Peggy was in school in the afternoon, Andrew and Annie took their naps. Dana and I walked out in the back yard together and looked for perfect fall leaves for her to bring inside and trace on pieces of white paper. As we walked she told me about her teacher and the names of her new little friends. She sat at the kitchen table with crayons or jars of finger-paints and traced on the pieces of white paper the fall leaves we had gathered. She colored the leaves in vivid shades of crimson and russet brown and golden yellow. She sang the little songs she learned in school softly to herself as she drew and colored. She was a shy little girl, patient and gentle with her younger brother and baby sister. When Andrew and Annie awoke from their naps, I brought them down to the kitchen to play on the kitchen floor while I made dinner or worked at my sewing machine. Dana got pots and pans out from under the kitchen cabinets, and I gave her potatoes to divide in piles. She taught Andrew the numbers she had learned in school by counting the potatoes as he put them into the pots. Then he recited the numbers on his own. He was a sturdy little boy, with ruddy cheeks and straight blond hair. Annie was a chubby, happy baby with a mass of dark curls and a Cupid's-bow mouth. Dana gently stopped Annie from trying to eat the raw potatoes and gave her a wooden spoon and her own pot to bang instead. When Peggy's bus was due, I'd put a gate up across the kitchen door and dash up the driveway to meet her bus and catch her as she jumped down.

Some days after school I put all the children into the car and drove into town to do the grocery shopping at the A&P. I carried Annie in one arm and took Andrew by the hand. The two older girls held on to the back pockets of my jeans, one on each side. In this way we crossed the parking lot into the store, like a floating "amoeba" as the grocery clerk always said. Some nights, on special occasions, I put the little ones to bed and let my older girls stay up later. Dana and Peggy and I watched the *Wizard of Oz* on television. I made popcorn and poured apple juice, and we watched the screen as the sky turned dark and Dorothy and Toto rushed for safety from the tornado whirling in the distance. My girls put their hands over their eyes at the sight of the Wicked Witch of the West, riding her bicycle into the wind outside Dorothy's window. "Ha, ha, ha, my pretty!" they shrieked. "I'll get you and your little dog, too!" Then they said along with the munchkins, "It's always best to start at the beginning! Get out of Oz altogether! Follow the yellow brick road!" Those were noisy, happy, hectic days with my little ones. I loved them.

I devoted myself to them. They were the reason for my marriage, my family. Harry worked two and three jobs to support us. I wanted them to be free of the fear and restraints of my childhood. And I wanted to give them, and Harry, the security he'd never had. Maybe that was the key to his heart . . . the reason for his distances? If he felt secure would he love me more?

My mother was never happier than in those days. My youngest brother was seven years older than Dana, and when he went to school my mother spent many of her days with my children. In the summers, she had them for weekends so they could spend days at the beach with her. She taught them card games and played checkers with them and taught them Parcheesi. She made little clothes for their dolls and taught them to shoot marbles. She bought them books and even more toys. She knit their sweaters and mittens and ski caps.

My mother and I took the little girls into New York before Christmas to see the *Nutcracker* ballet at Lincoln Center on the West Side. They wore matching blue-plaid coats and black velvet dresses with lace collars. They wore white tights and red patent leather shoes. We sat in the mezzanine and they stared in awe as the house lights dimmed and the orchestra began the overture to the ballet . . . that lovely, delicate music that is always so full of anticipation. Then the curtain opened, and a great Christmas tree rose, towering over the stage. After the ballet, we drove over to the East Side. We parked our car and walked down Fifth Avenue in the winter twilight. We stopped to look at the Christmas displays sparkling in the windows of Tiffany's and Saks Fifth Avenue. We walked across the avenue to the skating rink at Rockefeller Plaza and watched the skaters gliding in circles under the golden statue of Prometheus reclining above the rink and the giant Christmas tree that soared above the whole scene. For them, it was a magical city.

On the way back to our car, we always stopped at Saint Pat's. My little girls stared up, as I had years before, at the graceful twin spires of the cathedral, rising incongruous and medieval among the other towers of Fifth Avenue. We went inside to the dim hush of the great church, walked down a side aisle to the Lady Chapel so that my mother could light her votive candle in front of the white marble statue of the Blessed Virgin Mary.

As the children grew older, Harry spent more time with them. He took Andrew to basketball practice and on the bus with him when the basketball team played away-games. He drove the girls to the library and sat in the reading room waiting for them while they chose their books. But he never seemed comfortable with the children, as if he were afraid to be close to them and hold them and hug them. He treated them in the same way he treated me. He was kindly but removed. I was terrified they would feel unloved and lonely. I lavished affection and praise on them. I began to indulge them. I spoiled them.

At Christmas, we had the tallest tree I could find. Christmas morning was an orgy of toys, dolls, dollhouses, bicycles, crumpled wrapping paper and ribbon. One year, Andrew lost his new bicycle two days after Christmas.

"Where is it?" I asked him.

"If I knew it wouldn't be lost, Mom."

"Don't be fresh, Andrew. Please."

I bought him another one. He left that at a friend's house and forgot about it. When he remembered to go get it, it was gone. He wanted another one. Harry said no.

"All the other kids have one," I said. "How will he get around?"

"He'll walk. Maybe then he'll learn to respect his things."

"But it wasn't his fault!"

"He has to learn to be responsible for his actions."

"But he's only eight!"

I bought him another one.

As the years went on and the children grew older, I volunteered to drive everyone to the movies, to Little League practice, on field trips and to sleepovers with friends. I gave birthday parties and invited whole classes of children from their school.

Harry stayed at school most nights until seven o'clock. The children had their dinner before he came home. They would be bathed and in their pajamas, ready for bed. Harry's dinner would be warm on the stove. When he arrived, I left for the theatre.

Over the years I played every role I had time for. I played Desdemona in *Othello*, Katherine in *The Taming of the Shrew*. I played Olga in Anton Chekov's *The Three Sisters*, Catherine Sloper in *The Heiress*, Nurse Ratched in *One Flew Over the Cuckoo's Nest*. I played Stella in *A Streetcar Named Desire* and Alma in *Summer and Smoke*. But now I didn't need to lose myself in the lives of the characters I played onstage. And I didn't need approval. After all, I was a married woman. I was a caring, loving mother. I was behaving perfectly in the accepted way that was expected of the women of my generation. As a Catholic, I did as I was commanded.

I went to confession every Saturday afternoon and to Mass every single Sunday. I was my husband's wife, my children's mother and my mother's daughter. I did as I was told and tried to live up to everyone's expectations. I had to. I had to have approval. Not from a theatre audience; I had to have my family's approval. Theirs was the approval I craved. I went to the theatre now simply because I was lonely. I had friends there and a common interest. And since I went there at night when Harry and my children would be asleep, no one in my family seemed to mind.

And so our lives went on, Harry as private in his interests and pursuits as ever, and I escaping into the theatre at night to ease my loneliness. But around us, in those days, America was changing, convulsing. The safe certitudes of the forties and the fifties, of our young lives, were crumbling. John Kennedy was assassinated, then Martin Luther King Jr., then Robert Kennedy. Students rioted on campuses. Some were shot by National Guardsmen at Kent State University protesting a war that America would eventually lose.

Even the church was changing. The priest said Mass in English. Young men and women with long hair sat at the foot of the altar on Sunday, strumming their guitars and singing, "Kum Bay Yah." They wore love beads, tie-dyed T-shirts and bell-bottom jeans. The nuns sat self-consciously in their pews, embarrassed and newly released from their habits. Suddenly one Sunday, it was no longer a mortal sin to eat meat on Friday. I wondered what happened to all those souls who had for all those centuries? I missed the deep rumblings and the ringing peals of organ music when Mass was over. I missed the high clear sound of the girl's choir. I missed the soothing mystery of Gregorian chants and of High Mass sung in Latin.

But in the little town in western Connecticut, we were remote, removed from the change. I saw "hippies" on television. I heard about feminine liberation. The farm at Woodstock was just a few miles across the fields from us, but all I remember about that weekend in August 1969 was an unusual, long line of cars on the rural road into town that Saturday when I went shopping with my four children at the A&P, and we sang along with the song that was playing on the car radio, "Hey, mister tambourine man, play a song for me . . . in the jingle jangle morning I'll come followin' you." I only sang along. I would never have followed.

And some things remained absolutely the same. Catholic married women were still submissive to their husbands and to the church. We were captives, held without contraceptives and controlled by fear of hell. To even think of divorce was to veer into a dangerous, forbidden zone. Harry went as faithfully as I did to confession every Saturday afternoon and to Mass every Sunday. He seemed to rely more and more on the church and the Sacraments as he got older, as if he needed even more security than he had in his youth.

Always, I hoped for that one moment or gesture that would bring Harry and I together in the way that we had been before our marriage, when we had shared our thoughts and hopes and dreams. Always, I wondered if he was as lonely as I was. I searched for that one key to unlock the silence that he had closed around himself. But I never found it.

Some Catholic men believed that women were of two kinds: the Madonna or the harlot, Mary or Mary Magdalen. A man's wife could not be both. Who could have sex with the Madonna? He must find the harlot. How did Harry believe? I tried many times to ask him. He wouldn't talk about his thoughts. He refused to discuss sex. So I never knew.

Every so often I found myself staring at an obviously happy married couple. I saw a husband and wife sitting in the bleachers at a Little League game, his arm thrown carelessly over her shoulders. I saw a husband and wife sitting next to me in a pew in church, her hand resting on his knee. I saw a husband and wife in the row in front of me at the theatre, silhouetted against the movie screen, her head resting against his shoulder. I never talked about the desolation of my marriage with anyone. What would people think? Was Harry as lonely as I? When I asked he never answered.

And every so often, I would explode in some kind of irrational anger that shocked everyone in the house, most of all myself. My outburst would always be over some small thing, like a hairbrush missing from the downstairs hall table, the one I used to give my girls' hair one final brush before they ran out of the house for the school bus. Or someone leaving footprints on a rug I had just vacuumed. Or some friend canceling an afternoon visit. My children would stare at me, a disapproving look on their faces, as if I was behaving in an embarrassing manner. But disorder made me nervous. Free time frightened me. What would I do with it?

In 1973, when Annie, our youngest, started first grade, I decided to take a morning class in British poetry at a nearby college. When the class ended that semester, I enrolled as a full-time student. I was thirty-four. I decided to finish college and work toward a degree in English. It was a perfect routine. I left for school when the children did and came home just in time to meet their school bus in the afternoon.

In the next semester I took a course in education along with my English courses. I was realizing that if I graduated with a degree in English and education I might become a teacher. Then I could be home with my children and earn a living teaching a subject I'd always loved. I could help Harry with the mortgage and the bills. I could fill up the empty spaces in my life doing something real, worthwhile and challenging.

In the fall semester of 1975, I took a philosophy course called the Age of Enlightenment. I read the works of Rousseau and Descartes and Immanuel Kant, philosophers who argued passionately for the power of human reason against dogmatic authority. They argued that the Roman Catholic Church had suppressed free will and exercised its power by keeping its members ignorant, fearful and guilty. These philosophies were directly opposed to everything I had ever been taught as a Catholic. These were the very books I was forbidden to read at Albertus Magnus!

In the Dark Ages, I read, the Catholic priest held the power of learning over the simple, illiterate peasants because he could read and they could not. The ignorant peasant was the fearful peasant who needed the priest and the church to save his soul. The mightiest Catholic king could not go to heaven unless a Catholic priest absolved his sins. The supremacy of the pope and the power of the Catholic Church were absolute and universal. Anyone who challenged that power or the supremacy of the pope was burned as a heretic and damned for all eternity. The church held power over this world and the next.

But I was reading Immanuel Kant's *Metaphysics of Ethics* in which he stated his belief that reason is the final authority for morality, not blind obedience to some law or custom. "Sapere Aude!" he wrote. "Dare to know! Have the courage to use your own intelligence!" By the end of that course, my mind was spinning. I was exhilarated and euphoric with the freedom of the new ideas I was learning. I couldn't wait to go to class every day. I'd made the dean's list every semester and won a scholarship in my last year at the college. For the first time since I was a girl, I began to see the possibility of my own freedom. I began to wonder about the possibility of getting a divorce. If I earned my own living, I could support my children by myself. But I dismissed the notion every time I thought about it. I could never break up my family.

That same spring, I accepted the role of Maggie in *Cat on a Hot Tin Roof*. I hadn't acted in several years. The director, a friend of mine, had always wanted to direct the play and he'd hounded me for years to take the role. I'd always put him off. I wasn't sure I could play Maggie, the "cat" of the title. The character is the sexually starved and emotionally frustrated wife of a former college football star. She spends most of the play trying to seduce her husband, who refuses to have sex with her or even to love her.

I'd always played fragile women, easily broken, lonely women who lived in their dreams and who had retreated from a harsh world into fantasy. But now I'd moved out of fantasy, away from fragile people. And the theatre was no longer important to me as it once had been. Now I wanted to play this character. I thought that this was a woman who took control and eventually got what she wanted. Something about the character of Maggie drew me to her: She was a fighter. I wanted to know how that felt.

Somehow, between classes, I learned my lines. I brought my homework to rehearsals. But when the play opened, I found myself waiting for the night when it would close. I was finding the theatre less interesting, claustrophobic and static. I was tired of repeating other character's lines and manufacturing emotions. It was no longer enough to fantasize, to get inside another character's skin. I wanted to be free, to live a real life with real challenges, real risks and real gains. In my excitement and anticipation, I never realized I might fail.

As Maggie, I spent the entire first act onstage in a white satin slip. For the second and third acts I wore a clinging dress of soft, cream-colored lace. The dress was a stunning creation, glamorous, sensual and elegant, cut low in front and made to fit close to my body. It was designed for seduction. I didn't realize how my new schooling was liberating me. I wore the dress as an affirmation of sex, not as a plea for it.

Some of Harry's friends and their wives saw me in the play and commented about the dress to him afterward. One night, halfway through the run, he was waiting up for me when I got home. I was surprised to see him sitting in the dining room so late at night. He wondered why I had to appear in front of people dressed in an alluring lace dress.

"What difference could that possibly make to you?" I said.

"Phil Gallagher said you looked very sexy in that dress."

"Good," I said. "That's how Maggie is supposed to look. She's trying to seduce her own husband." I walked past him on my way upstairs.

"I don't think the kids want to go to school and have their friends say you are parading around in a dress like that," he said.

"It's a play," I said. "Besides, I don't care what a bunch of kids say." I started up the stairs.

"Well, then maybe you should think about how I feel," he said.

I stopped on the stairs

"How do you feel? I never know."

"I don't want to hear this," he said.

I came down the stairs and walked over to him.

"Why did you bring it up then?" I said. "How do you feel?" I saw that he wasn't going to say anything.

"Answer me!" I said. "How do you feel?" I didn't realize I was screaming at him until he jumped up and grabbed my arm.

"Answer me!" I screamed.

He didn't answer. He slapped me across my face. Blood poured out from my nose. He turned and left the house. I heard his car start, pull out of the garage and drive away. I listened for sounds of my children awake, but I heard nothing. Then I went into the downstairs bathroom and washed the blood from my face. My hands were shaking. I sat down quietly in a dining room chair. Why did he do it? Had he just noticed that I had changed? Was he suddenly aware that I had made a life of my own? What did he care? He couldn't answer and I had no more interest in asking. I didn't care what he thought anymore. I felt nothing. And that complete absence of feeling frightened me more than anything ever had. That was the night I knew I would end my marriage.

I finished the play. I wore the lace dress. I finished the semester and signed up for a full load of summer courses. I avoided Harry, except to tell him that I would be taking summer courses and that I wanted him to be at home with the children on those mornings since he wouldn't be teaching. We were polite as always. But my marriage was over. I was deeply afraid my children knew what had happened between their father and me, that they'd overheard our argument. But I didn't want to talk about it for fear they didn't know. Instead I kept up the charade of a marriage for their sake. It was easy. I'd had years of practice. But the growing distance between their father and me was obvious.

I was preoccupied, nervous and rushed in the last months of college. I threw myself into my courses because I wanted the best possible teaching job when I graduated. I did my student teaching at Staples high school in Westport. I taught all day, took two required courses after school, then rushed home and prepared lesson plans for the next day.

My children picked up on my tension. They were miserable. Dana began to clean compulsively. She lost her temper if anyone came down after supper for a snack and disturbed the kitchen. One night I found her wiping the refrigerator door, over and over, with Windex and a piece of paper towel. A pile of used paper towels was at her feet. She went over the same spot on the door, her eyes so fixed on it that she didn't see me standing there watching her.

"Dana, stop," I said.

"It isn't clean! It isn't clean!" she cried. I put my arms around her.

"It doesn't have to be that clean," I said. "Just leave it alone. I'll do it."

One afternoon Peggy moved out of the bedroom she shared with Dana. Peggy had laid her school clothes out on her bed that morning and gone into the bathroom to brush her teeth. While she was gone, Dana hung the clothes back up in the closet. Dana hounded her about any disorder, including pencils and books that were not in neat piles on her desk, shoes left on the floor or her bed not made as soon as she got up. Peggy went silently up and down the stairs carrying armloads of her clothes and books and brought them into the living room. She got the pillows, sheets and blankets from her bed and arranged them on the living room sofa. She put her record player on the floor next to the sofa and began to play Elton John's "Daniel" over and over again.

"Peg," I said. "Can't you talk to Dana about this? Tell her to stop touching your things."

"Do you expect her to listen to me, Mom? She doesn't stop when you tell her."

Andrew spent all his time with his friend Tim, fishing at the lake near our house. When he came home he rode his bicycle recklessly down the driveway and jammed on the brakes so that gravel spun up around the wheels. He couldn't sleep some nights, worried about his health. He feared his heart would beat too fast and that he would be stricken with a heart attack in the night. Nothing I said could ease his worry.

One week Annie missed three days of school. The day she went back I got a call from her teacher. Would I see her after the school day? She was concerned about Annie.

"Your daughter is angry that the class has gone on without her. She is disturbed that the others have learned something she did not."

"Oh?" I said. "Well I'm sure she'll catch up."

The teacher stared at me.

"I don't think you understand the problem here," she said. "Annie thinks the world revolves around her. She is very upset to think that it does not. She expected that class would stop when she wasn't here." The teacher hesitated. "She appears to be spoiled."

The teacher was right. All my children thought that the world revolved around them because at home, with me, it did. I was trying, desperately, to make their world as normal as I could for as long as I could. But it was as if my children sensed what was coming and in desperation asked me for more and more security when I had none to give them.

I made an appointment with a psychologist who specialized in family therapy. I insisted that Harry come with the children and me. They sat silently, looking bored and distrustful in the therapist's office.

"Well," said the therapist. "Let's start with Andrew. Why did you want to come?"

"I didn't," said Andrew. "My mother made us."

"Why do you think she wanted you to come?"

"I don't know."

"Andrew," I said. "You worry about your health! You don't sleep! Why?"

"I'm not talking about that here," said Andrew. "It's none of his business."

The therapist turned to Dana.

"Anything you'd like to discuss?" he said.

Dana shook her head no.

"Peggy?"

"No."

I insisted that we go back to the therapist three times. At the end of the third session the psychologist said, "It's difficult to be a family if none of you speak."

"Can't we just go home?" said Annie.

On the way home Harry said, "What a waste of time and money."

They all refused to go back. I went alone several times and stopped. What was the point?

Several months later, on a Saturday morning, I was alone in the house. I had just graduated from college. Harry was coaching at school and the children were all with friends. I was vacuuming the living room rug. I started at the doorway and went back and forth, vacuuming the rug in long stripes until I reached the far corner of the room. I stood there and looked back across the room at the pretty, alternating bands of light and dark gold on the rug. I was pleased at the orderly rows. But I couldn't get across the room to the door without leaving my footprints on the neat, clean design I'd made. I couldn't make a mess in the perfect world I was trying to create. So I sat down in the corner. I heard Annie come down the hall. She looked in at me from the doorway.

"Mom, what are you doing?" she asked.

"I don't know," I answered.

CHAPTER FIFTEEN

A Dream of Women Cut in Half

In the days and weeks before I told Harry I wanted a divorce, I looked feverishly for a teaching job. I applied to several area high schools, but the job I wanted was at Choate Rosemary Hall, an elite prep school in Wallingford, Connecticut. I had met the dean of faculty some months before, a silver-haired man in his early sixties who wore old snow boots, rumpled khaki pants and a baggy maroon sweater. He welcomed me into his book-lined office where a cheerful fire snapped in the fireplace. I'd told him that my plan was to live on campus with my children and teach there until I retired. He told me that teachers at Choate taught a full load of classes and coached a sport after school. Some teachers lived in the dormitory with the students. Would I be able to relocate, he wondered. Would my husband consider a teaching job as well? Now I called the dean of faculty and asked him if there were any openings. A senior English teacher was thinking about retiring, he said, but he would have to let me know.

I couldn't sleep at night. Stomach cramps seized me in the middle of the night. I paced the house in the darkness and stared out at the expanse of lawn and the grove of white birch trees that Harry had planted years before. They looked still, ghostly in the moonlight. I looked down the long driveway to the white gate at the end. The leaves of the birch trees stirred and threw moonlit-shadows on the gate. What was I about to do? Was there any way to avoid it? Who could I ask? Who could I tell? No one but Harry.

One night we drove to the movies and parked outside. I told him then that I wanted to leave him. I told him in the car, in the darkness of the parking lot. He stared straight ahead, his hands resting on the steering wheel.

"I don't blame you," he said, without expression. "I knew this was going to happen. I haven't been a very good husband."

I had half expected that he would argue with me or make some small protest. But he didn't. He seemed somehow relieved. Tired. It was as if he had finished fighting a long, secret battle and he could finally rest.

"We should see a priest," he said. We drove home and I called the same priest who years before as a young curate had comforted me and arranged for our marriage. We'd been friends for years. He'd come to visit me in the hospital after the birth of each child, baptized all of them, and come to our house for dinner and holidays. He had his own parish now, close to where we lived. He wasn't surprised to hear what I told him.

"You and Harry should come in separate cars," he said. "I'd like to talk to you alone afterward."

Harry and I arrived at the rectory several nights later. We went into his office.

"Is there any hope of saving this marriage?" he said.

He looked at Harry then at me. He was a big man, burly and fleshier with the years.

"No," I said. "None."

The three of us talked briefly. Of course I realized I could not receive the Sacraments . . . unless our marriage could be annulled. Harry took the address of the Bishop's office.

"How long does an annulment take?" he asked.

"I can set everything in motion soon," said the priest.

He saw Harry out and then came back into the office and sat down next to me.

"I'm sorry that you and Harry have decided to part," he said.

"It wasn't a very happy marriage," I said.

"Why did you have sex with him?"

"Father," I said, "you should know the answer to that. Catholic wives aren't supposed to deny their husbands."

"Did you love him?"

"Yes."

"Did he love you?"

"I don't know," I said. "He never said he didn't love me."

"But did he tell you that he did?"

"Before we were married he told me all the time. After we were married he never told me anymore. Never." Tears filled my eyes.

He put his arm around me as if to comfort me the way he had years ago when we sat together in the dark, old church when I was nineteen and pregnant and alone. He leaned close to me and put his hands up to my cheeks as if to brush my tears away.

"You need someone to love you," he said. "You have been lonely for too long." He took my face in his hands and leaned closer to me.

"Oh, Father," I said. "I can't even think about someone loving me. I have to think about what I'm going to do now. I . . ."

He pressed his lips on my mouth. I put my hands against his chest and tried to push him away from me, but his hands on my face were too strong. He ran his tongue along my lips and tried to force it into my mouth. I was shocked at how practiced he was, how insistent. I was afraid of him.

"Stop!" I gasped. "Get away from me!"

"But I love you," he said. "I've been in love with you for years."

"You took vows!" I said.

"So did you," he said.

"You're a priest!" I screamed.

He put his finger across my mouth.

"Sssh," he said. "I'm a man, too."

"No!" I screamed. "It's not fair!"

I shoved him away and ran out of the rectory. I ran to my car and drove home. I burst in on Harry, watching television.

"The priest tried to kiss me!"

"Susan, calm down," Harry said. "He's a man, too, you know."

෧ඁ෧ඁ෧ඁ

Our youngest daughter, Annie, screamed when we told her we were getting a divorce—"Nooooo!"—a terrible, piercing cry. She threw her hands up to her ears as if to block out the words she had just heard. "No!" She was ten.

Andrew was twelve. He stood in front of us and shook his head silently back and forth. Tears spilled down his cheeks. He tried to wipe them away quickly, first with one hand then the other, but he couldn't. They came too fast. He covered his face and sobbed.

"Oh, no," he kept saying. "Oh, no."

Dana, sixteen, said quietly, "I knew it," and then sighed as if relieved of a great burden she had carried for too long. She went out into the hallway where Peggy was waiting.

"It's over," she told her.

Peggy came in and stood in front of us and listened as we told her that we couldn't continue to be husband and wife but that we would always be their parents. When we finished, she stared at Harry for a very long moment. She said nothing. Then she looked at me. Her eyes were empty as if drained of all feeling. She was fifteen. She turned abruptly and left the room. She did not speak of the divorce to anyone. Not to me or her father or her grandmother or to any of her friends. Her best girlfriend didn't learn of it until a year later, well after the divorce was final.

That night, after the children had gone to bed, Harry and I sat down at the dining room table.

"I can't afford to move out. I'll never be able to pay the mortgage here and a rent for myself somewhere else," he said.

"We'll have to sell the house," I said.

"You want to put these kids through that, too?"

"We both agreed on this divorce," I said.

"You're the one who wants it," he said. "I don't want it. It's a mortal sin."

"What should I do?"

"You're the one who wants this," he said again. "I think you should go. You can find work."

"But I can't leave them!"

"They'll be fine with me for a while. As soon as you're on your feet you can take them with you. Then we'll sell the house and you can buy your own."

"I don't know what I'm doing!"

"I know," said Harry. "That's why they're better here with me for now." He paused for a minute. "Because I think you're unraveling. And I can't help you. I don't know how."

~~~~~

I waited to tell my mother about the divorce until the last possible moment—the day the legal notice of it was filed in the *Bridgeport Post*. It was a Saturday morning. I drove to Fairfield at eight o'clock in the morning and found my mother and father in the kitchen having their tea. I told them that Harry and I were getting a divorce. My mother was disbelieving.

"No. No," she said to me. "You can't." Then she looked at my father. "Tell her she can't!"

My father glanced up at me. He got up, crossed in front of me with his cup and saucer, and put them in the sink.

"I can't tell her anything," he said and left the kitchen.

"What will happen to the children?" she asked.

"They'll be safe."

"What will you do?"

"Teach."

"Where?"

"I don't know yet."

"Why did this happen? Why didn't you ever say how unhappy you were?"

"Because it wouldn't have mattered. Anyway, it was my business."

On the day I left, Peggy came to me as I was putting my things in the car. I had found a place to stay temporarily, with four friends in Wilton several miles away.

"Mom, can I come with you?" she asked.

She began to cry for the first time. She looked at me with her clear, pale eyes. I saw her again as the infant in my arms on the day she was born when she'd gazed up at me with so much trust and wonder in those eyes. Now they were filled with anguish and a terrible sorrow. I put my arms around her and kissed her.

"I can't take you with me now, Peg. As soon as I'm settled you'll come with me. It's only for a little while."

When would I be settled? Where? I had no idea. How could I take her when I didn't know where I was going?

I drove to the house in Wilton, a big old farmhouse at the end of a quiet, tree-lined road. It had five bedrooms and three bathrooms. Four friends of mine rented it. A married couple, both high school teachers; a young woman; a graduate student in psychology; and an actor friend of mine from the community theatre who was starting a professional career in New York.

I spent those first days and weeks looking frantically for a teaching job. I drove to every high school in the area and had interviews with every high school principal. But it was October, and positions were all filled. I called Choate and badgered the dean of faculty. The teacher I was to have replaced had decided not to retire. "Maybe next year," the dean told me. "Keep in touch." The only work I could find was as a substitute teacher for twenty-five dollars a day. Some weeks I worked four days. Some weeks I didn't work at all. I had no money. Though my lawyer begged me to take alimony, I refused it. Harry had said he couldn't afford it. "Any money I have to give you will come out of the children's mouths. Besides, you can work. They can't."

I drove over to see my children every day. At night I fell into an exhausted sleep. But every night I had the dream. The yellow school bus rolling up to the door of the vacant house. My children's anguished faces framed in the back window of the bus. The bus rolling away from me. Every night I woke crying, sometimes screaming. One night, Tom, the actor, and Rebecca, the student, came in to my room and sat down next to me on the bed.

"What is it, Susan?" she asked.

"What have I done?" I cried. "My children! My kids!"

"You're going to make yourself sick," she said. "You can't go on like this. Go back to the house and tell Harry he has to leave."

"I can't!" I said. "He won't be able to support them! How can I support them? I can't support myself!"

"Whose idea was this that you should be the one to leave?"

"His."

"It's wrong. He'll have to do it," she said.

"He says he can't! He says this is best for them! I have to find work. I have to!"

Tom took my hand. "Susan, calm down," he said. "I have an idea that might help. We'll talk about it tomorrow. Try to sleep."

The next morning he told me his plan. I would go into New York with him and meet his agent. She would send me out on auditions for television commercials. One commercial would pay me residual money every time it was shown.

"I don't want to be an actress," I said. "I'm a teacher."

"You don't have to be an actress," he said. "All you have to do is spend one day making a commercial and then you get paid every time it runs. You get paid while you're looking for other work."

I took the train into New York with him and met his agent. She sent me to meet a casting director who was looking for a "young, upscale, suburban, wife/mother type" for a coffee commercial. The casting director was also looking for an assistant. Her office was a madhouse. The waiting room was jammed with actors and actresses. She was talking on two phones at once behind her desk, then putting the people on hold while she rushed actors and actresses into her studio to videotape them as they read for the commercial. Glossy black and white pictures of actors and actresses were strewn all over her desk and in piles on the tables of the waiting room. I went in to read for the commercial.

"Thank you," she said. "That was very nice. I haven't seen you before. Are you new in New York?"

Her phone rang before I could answer.

"I'm sorry," she said.

"That's okay," I said. "Don't you have anyone to help you?"

"No," she said. "Do you know anyone who needs a job?"

"Yes," I said. "I do."

"Why would you want to work for me?" she said. "You could do very well making commercials."

"I'm not an actress," I said. "I don't have any time for make-believe. I need something real that I can count on."

Three days later the agent called to tell me I had the part. I went back into New York and filmed the commercial. Then I went to work for the casting director that winter. I drove from Wilton to Stamford very early every morning and took the eight A.M. train into the city. I worked until six at night and sometimes later. One night in January we worked until eight o'clock taping children for a toy commercial. The casting director asked me to hand-deliver the videotape to the commercial's director at his Madison Avenue office on my way to catch the train at Grand Central Station. Our office was on the West Side of the city just off Broadway. I rushed across town, delivered the tape and then hurried down Fifth Avenue toward the station. It was bitter cold. The wind whipped up the avenue, sending pieces of paper and other trash dancing and twirling before it. Dust and dirt and the cold wind stung my eyes as I ran down the avenue.

I missed the nine o'clock train. I sat down on one of the wooden benches in the waiting room to wait until the next train at ten. All around me on the other benches were the homeless, some sitting slouched down, some staring vacantly, some sprawled out on the benches with mouths open snoring. The waiting room stank of urine. I remembered the days when I had rushed through this waiting room in my school uniform to change my clothes in the ladies room and then meet my friends. Then the floors and benches were polished until they shone and the ladies room was spotless and smelled of clean soap and expensive perfume.

The train arrived in Stamford at eleven o'clock that night. It was bitter cold, and the train station was deserted. I got into my car and turned the key in the ignition. Nothing happened. I tried again. There was only a faint clicking sound in the car. The battery was dead in the frigid cold. I hired a cab to get to Wilton. The ride cost twenty dollars in addition to my train fare. I made only seventy-five dollars a week. I received residual checks for the commercial, but I never knew when a check would come, and when one did, it was never for more than a few hundred dollars. Most of the money I made I spent on the train fare back and forth to the city.

I saw no alternative but to move to New York. I left the car in Connecticut and moved into the city. I sublet cheap apartments from actors who went out of town for months at a time with touring companies or to work in regional theatres. When one actor returned to New York, I moved to another apartment. Alone at night in the strange apartments the reality of what I had done overwhelmed me. I was powerless to escape my guilt. I was tormented by the loss I had caused my children. It didn't matter that they were safe in the house with their father and that I talked to them almost every day and saw them every weekend. I was not there. I pushed my tears down so that my throat ached. I dared not allow myself to cry. If I did, I thought I would never stop. The days became like the nights, colorless, hollow periods of time that I prayed would pass until the weekends came and I could see my children.

A driving snowstorm descended one weekend that I'd promised to see them. I took the train out of New York, picked my car up at the station and drove through the storm to see them. They looked at me as if wondering what I was doing there and why I came. That spring Harry sold the house. I gave him my share of the profit for the down payment on another smaller house that he'd found for himself and the children.

Peggy called me in New York several weeks before one of the big dances at her high school. She had seen me in the lace dress I'd worn as Maggie in *Cat on a Hot Tin Roof,* the last play I'd done, and she wanted to wear the dress to the dance. I thought it strange that Peggy would want to wear a very elegant and alluring dress that I'd worn in a play.

"Why do you want to wear that dress, Peg? You're only sixteen. Isn't it a little old for you?"

"I'm sure it will fit, Mom."

"I know it'll fit, but aren't you too young to wear it?" But she insisted.

I went up to Connecticut and got the dress out of my mother's attic. On the Friday night of the dance, I drove back and helped her get ready. The dress did fit her perfectly, but she seemed awkward in it as if it was a beautiful dress of mine that she had wanted but didn't know how to wear. I thought she was trying to be like me but somehow not getting "me" right. And she was so young!

She was a superb student. She was secretary of her class and homecoming queen. She loved organizing parties for her friends and she was busy with them almost every weekend. One weekend she came into New York. She loved the city. I was working that Saturday morning in the casting office, trying to tidy some of the mess of the past week. She helped me put actor's pictures in neat piles according to types: children, cute, mop-tops; children, preteen, serious; young, suburban dads, mid thirties; older men, distinguished, spokesmen; young suburban moms, mid thirties; and older, upscale women, forties, spokeswomen; teen-age girls, all-American. These were girls of Peggy's age, sixteen, with round faces and not yet matured into the gaunt angles and pronounced cheekbones of later years when they would all be watching their weight too closely. We'd had twenty or so girls in the day before to read for a commercial for Quaker Oats cereal. I saw her looking at their resumes, the lists of commercials each had done, which were stapled onto the backs of the pictures.

"Are these girls really just sixteen?" she asked.

"Yes," I said. "They can earn quite a nice living doing these commercials."

"If I made commercials, that would help with my college tuition," she said.

"That's true," I said. "But you're going to a state university. Your tuition won't be that much."

She picked up a script for the commercial.

"Can I try reading this?"

"Sure," I said. "I'll videotape you just for fun, and you can see how you did."

She stood in front of the camera and read the lines of the commercial with such ease and sincerity that I was astonished. She spoke into the camera as if to someone she had known all her life. At the end of the last line, she gave a small, impish grin as if sharing a charming secret with the camera and then she laughed.

"How was I?" she said.

"You were terrific," I said.

"Do you think I can audition like these girls?"

"Absolutely," I said. "But wait till you graduate. You always tell me how much you love school. As soon as you finish, you can do what you want. I'll help you. I can introduce you to all the agents."

That night she helped me move from one apartment to another sublet, this one a walk-up on West Seventy-sixth Street just off Central Park. It poured rain. We sloshed through rainwater up to our ankles, dragged several sodden cardboard boxes out of the car and lugged them up five flights of stairs. Peggy laughed and chattered all the way up and down those stairs, I thought to keep my spirits from sagging. I didn't want her to know how depressed I was at the thought of living in yet another sublet—some other person's home— so I laughed and chattered along with her. Just before we got into the car to drive back to Connecticut, she stood and turned her face up to the rain. She looked at the streetlights and the glistening pavements and the lights of the avenue that runs along Central Park.

"I love this city," she said. "One day I hope I live here." I remembered myself at her age and the dream I had lost.

I wanted her to have her dream. I showed the tape to the casting director the next Monday. "You're right," she said. "She's a natural."

But my other children were silent, sad and removed when I saw them. When I was with them I tried to anticipate their wishes. I tried to cater to every whim. I tried to explain away every problem, sympathize with any hurt. I never said, "no," or "you are wrong." How could I say that to any of them?

As the months passed, I felt helpless to change the course I had set for myself. Were my children as heartbroken as I? What had I done? How could I have hurt so many people? Then my mother died.

She was never as robust as she looked. She'd always been fragile and frightened. She had been devastated by my divorce. I had destroyed her vision of family and her reputation, the only security she had ever known. She resigned from the Ladies Guild at the church. She stopped playing bridge with her friends. She even avoided her sisters. She felt obliged to explain what I had done, but she couldn't. She couldn't understand it. She was mortified.

She began to complain of a pain in the upper part of her back so she saw her doctor who referred her to the hospital for x-rays and tests. She was diagnosed with a malignant tumor in her right lung. The cancer was aggressive. I went back to the house to help my father and my sister and brothers take care of her. In that short, futile time, she lost the little strength she had left. One afternoon I sat next to her, close to her on her bed, I held her in my arms. She was very weak and drugged, and she could only whisper to me.

"Do you know how the thread spins out on my sewing machine?" she asked.

"Yes," I answered.

"That's what my life is doing." Then she looked up at me with a strange, sweet half-smile. "It's out of my hands."

She died a week later. She died just before dawn on a cold, gray November morning, forty years to the day after her father. My father and my sister and I drove, through a light snow that had fallen in the night, to the hospital and walked through the dim, silent corridors to her room. My mother lay as if sleeping under the white hospital sheets. How could she be so still? My sister and I were stunned at the silence. We were beyond tears. My father looked at us, questioning. "Should I kiss her?" he asked. We didn't know how to answer.

My mother's coffin, draped in a simple white satin cloth, embroidered with a gold cross, lay at the foot of the altar in the old church. My children sat in their pew and stared at it silently as a priest circled it and blessed it with holy water. "We are poor, banished children of Eve, sending up our sighs, mourning and weeping from this valley of tears. Margaret, you have sacrificed in this life so that you will be happy in the next," he said. "May the angels take you into paradise; may the martyrs come to welcome you on your way." The organist played my mother's favorite hymn to the Blessed Virgin Mary.

Mother dear, oh pray for me,
While far from heaven and thee,
I wander in a fragile boat
O'er life's tempestuous sea.

She had always thought of herself as helpless. When her funeral mass was over, my bewildered children followed her coffin out of the church. A light snow was falling. She who had held them when they were tiny infants, who had read *Stuart Little* and *James and the Giant Peach* when they were too young to read for themselves, who knit mittens and red sweaters and long Christmas stockings with their names on, who taught them Parcheesi and let them stay up late on summer weekends, who had been with them for every birthday, every Christmas, every Easter and every day, was gone.

It was unbelievable to me that she could die and that I would never see her again or hear her voice. That I could never tell her I loved her. How could I have disappointed her so profoundly? I was certain I had killed her. I believed she had lost her will to live and died because of the shame I had brought her.

My father went through the day of her funeral as if in a daze. Late at night after the friends and relatives who had gathered for her funeral had left, I found him sitting alone in the little room off the kitchen where my mother used to sew and watch television. The room was dark, and he was sitting in her rocking chair, rocking back and forth with his head to one side, staring into the darkness as if wondering what had happened to change his life so completely. Watching him, I thought of the losses my father had endured in his youth. What could it have been like for him in the visitor's room of that insane asylum, trying to understand where his father had gone even while he was staring into his father's vacant eyes? What could he say to his mother, what comfort could he have given her, on the way back to Queens on the bus? I understood that my father's house had always been the cornerstone, the anchor and the security of his life, but now my mother was gone from it. What would his life be like now, without his wife, my mother? I had no idea. I went up to him in the darkness as he rocked in her rocking chair.

"Dad, are you all right?"

"Yes," he said without looking at me. "Thank you."

"Try not to worry about anything, Dad. We are all here to help."

"Yes," he said. "Good night."

"I'm sorry, Dad."

"Yes, I know." He stared into the darkness. "Good night."

My father left to spend several weeks with my mother's older sister and her husband in Florida. He called me in New York just before he was to return and asked me to close the house for the winter.

"Why, Dad? Don't you want to go home?"

"It isn't home."

I took the train up to Fairfield, drove to the house and went in. It was airless and dark. I remembered the house in the days when my mother was alive. Then it was always full of light. Plants bloomed on windowsills. Flowers filled the cut glass bowl on the dining room table. The clock sounded its soft chimes at every hour. Now the grandfather's clock that had been my grandmother's was stopped. The keyboard cover was pulled down tight over the piano keys.

I had gone back into New York after her funeral. At night I dreamed of women cut in half, sliced down the middle, still smiling, still walking, but not talking, both sides in perfect synchronicity as if they were still connected together. They had white faces and painted red lips like the mute characters in mime shows. I could never see their eyes. They had no breasts. I would wake, deeply fearful, and then suddenly remember that my children were lost and my mother was dead.

I felt a crushing, physical pain in my chest as if I couldn't breathe. Then panic. I had caused every sorrow my family was enduring. Wasn't I the selfish one who wanted the divorce? I had outlived my usefulness. I began to believe it was time for me to die, that it would be a relief to die. I was filled with a deep sense of dread. My fear was of breast cancer. I thought that should be the way I would die.

And now here I was, two years later, with the disease I had always dreaded. The hospital room was dark. The woman's husband was gone. She was sleeping. I looked again at the book in my lap: "The cancer patient seems to have been vitally dependent on other persons, other things . . . and when separated from those objects is lost. . . . We have found there has been a great mental suffering, a total destruction of hope . . . then trouble comes."

CHAPTER SIXTEEN

Forgiving Myself: Day Six

Dr. McCullough woke me the next morning.

"How are you?"

"Great."

"You look tired. Bad night?"

I couldn't think of what to tell him. What was I going to say? That I spent last night remembering the past twenty years?

"I'll sleep better when I'm home," I said. "When can I leave?"

He paused for a minute, and then he said, "When we did the mastectomy, we took some lymph nodes out from under your arm."

"Yes?"

"We sent them to be checked, and we don't have the results back yet."

"Tested for what?"

"We want to be sure the cancer didn't spread to those."

I was stunned. I was over cancer! Wasn't I? What was my body doing to me?

"What does it mean?" I said. "Can't I go home?" I could hear my voice shaking.

"Not yet," he said. "They're still checking."

"Oh," I said.

I couldn't think of anything else to say. I stared at him. He couldn't think of what to say either. He stared back at me as if trying to understand what I was thinking. He was a gentle person. He didn't have the obvious, high energy of Dr. Siegel. He had a deep calm, a quiet kindness. "I'll let you know just as soon as we find out," he said. "Try not to worry." And he went out. I didn't have the strength to worry. I felt shocked. Helpless. Exhausted.

A short time later Dr. Siegel came in. "How are you?"

"I don't know." I said. "I'm scared. I thought I was okay." I told him about the lymph nodes.

"Remember, you're in charge here," he said. "Remember what I told you about the seat belt? It's important to feel in control."

"I want to be in charge," I said. "But I'm really scared. It's hard to feel in control when you're sitting in a hospital bed, bandaged up and attached to these tubes." I waved my left hand at him with the IV line stuck in it.

"A hospital is a great practice ground," he said. "If you can feel in control of yourself in here, just think how powerful you'll feel when you get out. If you look at something that happens to you in here and you say, 'I can't change this,' that's when you start feeling helpless and fearful. That's not good for your body. But if you say, 'This event is not in charge, I am,' that's the first step toward using your own power and you stay calm."

"If only they could study emotions under a microscope," I said. "Like my lymph nodes!"

"Listen," he said. "The body can reflect the mind. It responds to what the mind is thinking. You could look on this concern as a way to become even stronger."

"I read the Simonton book you gave me. I don't want to see things as hopeless. I don't want to feel helpless."

"Illness isn't your failure. It can be a way of changing your life. Did you ever think that this whole experience could be changing your life in a very meaningful way? It's how you look at it." He stared at me with a knowing look. "I can see you have the spirit to try to figure yourself out. The mind and the spirit can heal the body. Don't forget the spirit." He patted my foot for emphasis.

Pat had been waiting out in the hall. Dr. Siegel saw him.

"Come on in," he said. "I'm Bernie Siegel."

"How are you?" said Pat.

"Wonderful," he said. Turning to me, he added, "Do your visualizations. See you later." He went off on the rest of his rounds.

"What are visualizations?" asked Pat.

"They're mental exercises," I said. "You visualize yourself getting well again."

"Are you doing them?"

"No," I said. "The cancer might be in my lymph nodes."

"What are lymph nodes?"

"They're glands. If the cancer went into them, then it probably spread all through my body."

"Well, do they know that? Did they tell you that?"

"They're still checking."

"So you don't know."

"No."

"So why aren't you doing those visualizations?"

"Why bother?" I asked.

Pat dropped the newspaper he was carrying on my bed.

"Here," he said. "I'm leaving."

"Why?" I said. "You just got here!"

"You Irish are in love with your sorrows. You are too damned depressing."

"I am not in love with my sorrows!"

"You're a fucking crepe hanger."

"What is a crepe hanger?"

"You see the world draped in black. Nobody's sorrows are worse than yours. You hang black crepe on everything."

"I do not!"

"Oh, yes you do. You refuse to think ahead. You want to bury yourself in your past. Well, go ahead. Bury yourself." And he walked out.

I hadn't noticed that Rita had overheard the whole argument. I put my head in my hands and started to cry.

"How could he be so unfeeling?" I cried.

"He loves you," she said simply. "And he's right. Remember what Bernie told you. It's how you look at things. You're not helpless."

"But I have this terrible scar! And I might not be over this damned thing!"

"You want to know what I think about that scar?" said Rita. "You got a second chance. That's how I see it."

Cancer is a symbol, as most illness is, of something going wrong in a patient's life. A warning to take another road. Was I missing a signal somewhere? Was this a sign that I needed to see things in a new way? Was the scar on my chest a symbol of a new life beginning? Or was it too late for me?

"It's how you look at things," Rita said. "You are not helpless."

You are important, said Dr. McCullough. *You have a choice,* said Pat. *Love yourself enough to protect yourself,* said Bernie.

All these people were telling me the same thing. Why wasn't I listening?

"You got a second chance," said Rita. A second chance for what?

I remembered when I thought my new life was beginning, just months before this day, on a Sunday afternoon in the early spring of

1979. I'd returned to New York after a weekend in Connecticut with my children. I was renting yet another sublet apartment, this one on the Upper West Side. As I stood in the Times Square subway station waiting for the subway uptown, a teen-age boy appeared out of nowhere and ripped my pocketbook off my shoulder. He ran away with it, down the platform and then up the subway stairs. I ran after him up the subway stairs and onto the street and the trash and crowds of Times Square. He had vanished into the crowd with every bit of money I had in the world; seventy-two dollars and my driver's license. I had no credit cards. I had no collateral.

I walked the thirty blocks uptown and up the five flights of stairs to my apartment. But it was not my apartment. I stood in the middle of it and looked around. It was another person's narrow, cluttered studio apartment, one room with a single window, crammed with another person's furniture and belongings. I had no furniture, no belongings except what was in my suitcase.

Suddenly I just got fed up, furious with the boy, furious with the damned city, furious with outside events and people like the boy ordering my life around, furious with myself for allowing all of it. I didn't have an epiphany. No great white light of understanding and revelation went off in my head. It was a commonplace, dirty event. People are robbed every day. Someone robbed me of something that was mine and I was sick of it. I wanted what was mine back. I was losing time with my children and going nowhere in a meaningless job in a godforsaken city. For what? Harry was in a house in Connecticut with my children. I was here. For what? I knew I would never allow my children to live in this city. It was a nightmare place. I would never bring them here. For some reason, standing in someone else's cramped little apartment, I finally realized my life belonged to me and I wanted it back.

I'd put my return ticket to Connecticut in the pocket of my jacket. Why? Coincidence? I called the casting director and told her what had happened and that I was taking the next day off. Then I called my father in Florida and asked him if I could stay for a while in the empty house. I already had the key. That was in my jacket pocket, too. I took my suitcase and walked back down to Grand Central Station. I left the city for good on the next train back to Connecticut. I commuted into New York for the next few weeks. I used the phone in the casting director's office to call every school principal within a twenty-mile radius of Fairfield. I called the dean of faculty at Choate and hounded him. He had to hire me, I told him. I was a perfect role model, a single working mother with four children. A month later, in March, the principal of a middle school in Easton, the town next to Fairfield, called me. The sixth-grade teacher was taking maternity leave. Would I like her job for the next three months until school ended in June? I accepted immediately and gave the casting director my notice. She begged me to stay.

Peggy had her heart set on becoming an actress, and I'd promised to introduce her to all the agents I knew as soon as she graduated. I told the casting director I'd continue to work for her on whatever weekends she might need me or whenever I had a school vacation. That way I could guarantee Peggy could meet those agents.

Two days after I started teaching at the middle school, I got a letter from the dean at Choate. I finally had the job I had been waiting for. Would I accept a position teaching in two departments? He realized it was lots of work, but I was well qualified to teach theatre arts as well as English. He hoped I would accept. Would I accept? Did he think I wouldn't? Was he crazy? Was he out of his mind? I was giddy with joy.

Just before Easter, the casting director frantically called me. She'd just landed an important contract, to cast the commercials for a big Coca-Cola campaign. She had to stay in New York to cast the principal actors for the speaking roles. Could I go to Fort Lauderdale to do the extra casting? The producers were looking for young men and women in their early twenties, tanned and athletic. She couldn't trust anyone else! Of course I would. I had to keep my hand in the business for Peggy.

I flew to Fort Lauderdale for Easter week and spent the days interviewing young local actors and actresses. In the early evenings, I sat next to the pool at a motel near the beach and watched the palm trees sway in the ocean breeze. The palm fronds made a soft, scraping sound as they rustled against one another. In the night sky, the white, moonlit clouds looked like the huge, billowing sails of tall old ships as they moved in off the ocean. It was, I thought, like paradise. It was the first time I'd been at rest for years. I looked forward to going back to my children, to my new job at Choate and my own home, and to what I thought was my new life.

I finished the school year at the middle school in June. Three weeks later, I met Pat. It was, I thought, the beginning of my new life. At least that's how I'd seen it. Then I got cancer. Now here I was in a hospital bed waiting to find out if the cancer was about to destroy me.

I thought of the quotation from the Talmud again: "We don't see things as they are. We see them as we are." I thought of my grandfathers. One lost his will to live; the other lost his mind. I thought of my mother, afraid of the loss of her good name and now dead like her father. They were all dead. *I can't be like them*, I thought. *I must change! How?* I remembered the boy stealing my pocketbook from me that Sunday afternoon in New York. In the end, he hadn't only robbed me of the only money I had left in the world. He robbed me of my inertia and helplessness and gave me back my will to live. I remembered Bernie telling me, "You have the spirit to figure yourself out. The mind and the spirit can heal the body. Don't forget the spirit." Now I understood that I had to find my own immune spirit, one that could withstand loss, overcome fear and overpower this disease. But what if it was too late?

I hadn't noticed that a man had come into my room and was standing next to my bed. He wore dark brown pants and a green shirt that looked like a Nehru jacket. He had a perfectly trimmed, short, light brown beard. A wooden cross hung from a gold chain around his neck. He smelled of some men's cologne that I couldn't place.

"Are you Susan Ryan?"

"Yes?"

He introduced himself as a Catholic priest, one of the hospital chaplains.

"Would you like to make a confession?"

I was living in sin. I was committing adultery with Pat. But to receive the Sacrament of Penance, to be absolved of my sin and avoid damnation, I had to promise never to commit the sin again. I had to promise never to see Pat again.

"No, Father," I said.

"I'm sure God will forgive you for any of your sins."

"That's between him and me," I said.

I remembered the priest who had blessed my mother's coffin. "Margaret, you have sacrificed yourself in this life so that you will be happy in the next," he'd said. My mother sacrificed her life for approval. She was dead. I'm not doing that, I said to myself. I don't care about approval. As the priest stood there watching me, the strangest thing happened. A quiet thing. A thought came to me, a remembrance from a gospel I knew almost by heart: "Not that we have loved God but that he has first loved us."

"I would encourage you to receive the Sacrament," said the chaplain.

"I'm not confessing anything," I said.

"The Sacrament is there to help you," said the priest. At that moment I understood that it wasn't. It had never helped me. It had terrified me and held me a fearful hostage. Suddenly I realized that beneath the layers of doctrine and dogma, fast days, feast days, holy days, votive masses, venial sins, extreme unctions, immaculate conceptions, litanies, processions, novenas, and penances, somewhere under all the words and rules and rituals was God. "God is there to help me," I said. "I'm going to forgive myself. Good night Father."

As he left, I thought, *I'm not on this earth to exist for other people and their approval. No. I'm here for me. I am not a bad person. I have a life to live and I will not die before I get a chance to live it.*

I lay quietly, closed my eyes and began my visualizations. I thought of my immune system as an army of little creatures dressed in white suits, massed together in front of me, waiting for me to give them the command to fight. "I'm in charge," I insisted to myself. "I'm in charge." I addressed the cells in my immune system. "Get going! Find those damned cells! Get them out of me!" I saw the little creatures surging through my body, searching for any dark, ugly cancer cells they came upon. "Fight!" I said to them. "Get rid of the damned things. You will not overcome me," I said out loud to the invisible cancer. "Get out. Just get the hell out. You die. I have a life to live."

At that moment, an absolutely amazing thing happened to me. I felt an instantaneous physical rush, a kind of flushing surge throughout my body. It was as if I could feel my "army" at work, as if my immune system had responded instantly to my command. I was astonished that I could do this thing. I couldn't get over it. The physical feeling was like a flood of warmth, almost electrical in its intensity. I knew then that my spirit was whole again. And then I experienced such a feeling of absolute well-being as I had never known. And then I fell sound asleep.

CHAPTER SEVENTEEN

A Sudden Freedom: Day Seven

The next morning I was awake for only a few minutes when Dr. McCullough rushed into my room. He looked stunned and disbelieving, as if he couldn't accept the reality of what he'd come to tell me. I felt a sinking feeling in my stomach when I saw his face. I prepared myself for what he was ready to tell me. *I'm in control,* I thought. *I will not lose hope. I will not be afraid. No matter what he tells me, I cannot afford to lose hope.*

"They're clear," he said.

"What?"

"There is no cancer anywhere. You're clear."

"What does it mean?" I couldn't understand what he said.

"You don't have cancer anymore. You're free." He looked at me strangely. "We were very worried about you. You were quite sick."

"Well, I'm not sick now," I said.

"I know. You're absolutely well." He seemed astonished.

"Thank you for everything Doctor," I said. "I'll probably never be able to thank you enough."

"You fought it," he said. "I watched you."

"Can I go home now?" I said.

"As soon as you'd like."

I was stunned. I called Pat at his office.

"Can you come pick me up?" I said. "I'm well. It's over. I want to go home."

"I'll be right up," said Pat.

Rita came in. "I'm supposed to unhook you from this IV," she said. She wore a huge smile.

"It's like a damned chain," I said. "Get me out of here."

"I'll see you in two weeks," said Dr. McCullough.

"Thank you for everything," I said again.

I rummaged around in my bag for my clothes. I put on a navy-blue sweater that buttoned up the front and a pleated skirt. I looked in the mirror at myself. I still had a bandage that covered the right side of my chest, but I looked flat on that side, lopsided. I took the sweater off and put my bra on loosely over the bandage. I could see the top of the red scar that ran down the front of my chest. That's okay, I said to myself. I got a second chance. I had an extra pair of knee socks rolled up in the bottom of my bag. I stuffed them into the empty place in my bra.

I saw the woman in the bed next to mine staring at me with a faint smile. "Necessity is the mother of invention," I said.

Bernie and Pat came in together.

"Well, look at you," said Bernie. "You're positively glowing!"

"You were right," I said. "Healing does happen from the inside out."

"I came to ask you if you want to join a new group that I'm forming called ECAP," he said. "It's for Exceptional Cancer Patients. I think you're one of them."

"Thank you, Bernie," I said. "But I never want to hear the word cancer again in my lifetime. Thank you so much for everything you told me."

"You listened," he said. "And then you changed." He looked at Pat. "You got a firecracker here," he said.

"Good," said Pat.

"Take care," I said to the woman lying in her bed. "Take care of yourself."

"Good-bye," she said.

I walked out of the hospital that morning into the clean, fresh November air and into my brand-new life. To this day, I can remember the sudden freedom of that morning. When I remember it I promise myself yet again never to waste a second of my life, never to lose the wonder of it—and never to live it for others.

On our way home in the car, Pat suddenly began to laugh hysterically.

"What?" I said alarmed.

"Oh, boy," he said. "The Big Fella is funny."

"Who?"

"God!" he roared. Tears of laughter streamed down his face.

"God?" I was still dazzled.

"Yeah! Aaaaah!" he wiped his eyes with the back of his hand as he drove. "What a sense of humor!"

"What are you talking about?"

"I've been a tit man all my life. Now look what God gives me. A smart-ass broad with one boob."

"So what if I only have one boob? Take it or leave it. I got a life."

"I know," he said, smiling. He looked over at me. "I can't even tell you how much I love you," he said.

I could see that my apartment was crowded with people as we pulled up outside.

"What's going on?" I said.

"Annie did it," said Pat. "She was so excited you were coming home that she told all the girls."

The girls greeted me with screams and laughter as we walked in. It was the Tuesday before Thanksgiving, and they were just out of school for the vacation. Many of their parents had come to pick them up, and they were crowded with their daughters into my apartment. All that afternoon other teachers from the faculty came and went, bringing sandwiches and cookies. The headmaster's wife came with an enormous basket of fruit and flowers. Toward early evening, the girls and their parents said their good-byes and left for vacation. I walked Pat out to his car.

"Will you be okay for the night?" he said. "I'll be back up tomorrow."

"Annie will help me," I said. "I'll be fine."

Sometime much later in the night, I woke. I heard a strange, persistent male voice coming from Annie's bedroom. The dormitory was deserted except for the two other teachers who shared dorm-mother duties with me, Monica and Beth. Monica's husband was on duty that night at Yale-New Haven Hospital. I went to the door of Annie's room and saw that a man was standing over her bed. He was small and dark with a goatee and stringy black hair. She lay there, petrified, staring up at him.

"What are you doing?" I said from the doorway.

I startled him. He turned from her bed and stumbled over to me. He was drunk and filthy and he stank of urine. He lifted his arm as if to strike me. I was bandaged from my shoulder all the way down to my waist and my right arm was in a sling.

All I could think of to do was to open my robe and scare him with my bandages. I did. He backed away from me so quickly that he fell on the floor. He crawled past me, like a crab, into the bathroom and knelt in front of the toilet bowl. He vomited into it and then sat back, exhausted on the bathroom floor. He swayed back and forth and then looked up at me as I stood in the doorway.

"You bitch!" he screamed. "See what you made me do? I'll kill you!"

"No, you won't," I said. "That would be stupid. Just get out of here and I won't call the police."

He got up and staggered out to the kitchen where he hung his head over the sink and retched into it.

"If you just get out of here, I won't call the police," I said again. I opened the front door to the apartment and showed him the darkness of the fields and woods that stretched beyond the parking lot of the dorm. "See?" I said. "You can leave. I won't do anything."

He staggered toward me and the front door. I stepped aside, and he fell out onto the front doorstep. I slammed the door behind him and rushed back to the door that led from our apartment into the common room of the dormitory. It was wide open. I could see through the common room to the front door of the dorm. That door was open as well. Someone hadn't locked it on their way out, and the security guard, on his rounds, hadn't noticed. I rushed out and slammed it shut. Then I went back into our apartment where I found Annie sitting in the kitchen. I called the police and the head of security at the school. Then I called Monica and Beth. I sat down with Annie in the kitchen.

"Well, that was exciting," said Annie, dryly.

"Not bad," I said. "I got him out, though."

When classes resumed after the Thanksgiving break I was determined not to let my students see any of my physical weakness. I didn't want them to be frightened. They were terrified of cancer, and they knew I'd had a mastectomy. I was the same age as their mothers, and this might frighten them even more. I wanted them to see that cancer was an illness I'd had that I didn't have anymore. It was over. I wanted them to see how normal I looked and how happy I was. So I stood facing them, holding a piece of chalk in my right hand like a sophisticate at a cocktail party, with my left hand cupped under my right elbow to support my arm. Then I turned around and began to draw diagrams of sentences on the blackboard, using my left hand to raise my arm as I drew. I drew diagrams of nouns and verbs and subjects and predicates, adjectives and prepositions and pronouns. Every day I forced my arm up and drew ever taller pyramids on the board on which sat gerunds and participles . . . ever more complex sentences until I could raise my right arm straight over my head.

I made myself walk down the hill to school every morning and back after classes to regain my strength, and I laid down and took a long nap in the afternoons whenever I was tired. I was determined to take care of myself, to understand what my body was asking me to do for it, to honor its requests.

The night before the Christmas vacation started, Annie and I walked down to the chapel for the annual candlelight Christmas Carol service. I wore an old fur coat, long and warm, that I'd bought in a thrift shop years before. Annie wore her favorite long black overcoat and a crimson, wool scarf. I looked at her in the glow of the candlelight as we sang the carols. She had a beautiful voice, high, clear and strong, like the peal of bells. She was becoming a young woman. I saw her dark hair massed in curls around the rose of her cheeks and her beautiful hazel eyes. I looked at Annie as if I'd almost lost her. She turned to look at me with a smile of absolute happiness. *Every second of life is so precious,* I thought. *How could I ever have wanted to escape it?*

Annie and I left the chapel and walked home across the campus. Snow had fallen earlier in the day and wrapped the place in quiet beauty. We walked past the old white colonial houses and saw through the windows the soft, warm lights of other faculty families. Fires blazed in their fireplaces and the smell of wood smoke hung in the cold air. As we came up the hill toward our apartment, I could see the glow of the old, brass hurricane lamp that had been my grandmother's in our window. Inside was my mother's gold and white brocade wing chair, my cherrywood dining room table and chairs, and my grandmother's tall clock. My mother had left it to me. It still chimed every precious quarter hour.

At the first faculty meeting after the Christmas break, I noticed some of the teachers staring at me as if surprised to see me. When I caught their eyes and smiled at them, they smiled back sadly as if resigned to some idea that I knew nothing about. They seemed frightened of me, as if I were different from them in some profound way. I wondered if they thought I was still sick.

Later, I told Pat how some of the teachers had looked at me.

"They probably are scared of you," he said.

"Why?"

"You've been someplace they haven't."

For weeks I wore a pair of rolled-up knee socks in the right cup of my bra. Two months after my mastectomy, I went into New Haven and bought a prosthesis, a small sack, the size of my missing breast, filled with liquid glycerine. When I got home, I put it in my bra and looked at myself in the full-length mirror. My hair was long and dark and my face was thinner, but there was color in my cheeks. Now I looked as though I had two breasts, but I was very thin, and I was shocked at how flabby my arms and legs had become. I called Pat.

"I'm too skinny and flabby. I want to be stronger. I have to be in control."

"Drive down to Fairfield," he said. "I'm taking you to my gym."

My day off from school was Friday. I drove down in the morning and met Pat outside the Iron Man Gym. I had never been to a gym in my life. I looked inside. Powerful-looking men stalked back and forth, posing in front of mirrored walls, puffing out their chests and flexing their biceps. I could see other men straining to lift heavy barbells. I peered through the window. I couldn't see any women inside.

"Come on!" said Pat. "What are you looking for?"

"I don't think this is for me, Patty," I said.

"What the hell are you talking about?"

"There are no women in there!"

"What do you care?"

I went in. I heard screams of pain and harsh, clanging noises as the men dropped heavy weights on the floor and slammed dumbbells back onto metal racks. It looked like a torture chamber and it smelled overpoweringly of sweat and iron.

"I can't do this," I said.

"Why?"

"I have nothing to wear."

"Yes you do," said Pat. He produced a pair of sneakers, shorts and a T-shirt.

"Where did you get these?" I said.

"I've been planning this for a long time." He smiled maliciously. "You might be forty, but you're not an old broad yet. Go in the locker room and change."

"There are men in there!"

"No, there aren't. I'll stand guard at the door. Get in there."

I went in and changed and came out into the gym. I was embarrassed standing there in shorts with my white flabby legs and arms in front of all the strange men. I worried that the prosthesis in my bra would fall out as I lifted the weight.

"Are you going to let that stop you?" asked Pat.

"No."

"Good. We'll start with legs! Legs! Legs!"

He was so enthusiastic. I did calf raises for my lower legs and leg extensions for my thighs.

"Good. Now stand over here," said Pat.

He stood behind me and placed a long, iron bar on my shoulders.

"What's that?" I said.

"Shut up and squat," he said.

"What?"

"Squat!"

"With this bar on my shoulders?"

"That's the point. You need to build strength in your legs. This is the way to do it."

I pushed myself through four sets of squats, excused myself, staggered to the bathroom and threw up in front of two huge men.

"Pain is gain!" they roared.

I staggered back out to the weight room.

"You've got flabby underarms," Pat announced. "Tomorrow we'll do six sets of French presses for your triceps and a shoulder routine."

I made myself go back the next day and did light arm and shoulder exercises. By Monday morning, every muscle in my body ached. I could hardly walk to my classroom, let alone write on the blackboard. But I made myself make the drive up and down to Fairfield three times a week to meet Pat at the gym. At the end of a month of this punishment, I began to notice subtle changes. I saw the faint definition of the muscles in my arms and thighs. They were firm, and they didn't wobble when I walked. And unbelievably, I felt energized, full of strength in spite of my aching muscles. The men were right. Pain is gain. Three months after my mastectomy I could lift a ten-pound weight with my right arm and raise it over my head—a victory sign!

I found the weight room in the Athletic Center at school, got up an hour early and worked out before class in the morning. I worked out for one hour every morning, five days a week. I worked upper-body muscles one day, leg muscles the next. I did 100 sit-ups after each workout. Weekends were free.

I learned patience and perseverance in the gym. Weightlifters and bodybuilders, like other athletes in training, know that strength is gained in months, not in days. I learned the importance of achieving small goals at first, on the way to bigger ones. Plutarch in the weight room: "Little by little!" I began to think about getting a breast implant. Pat was excited for me.

"There's plenty of time for that," he said. "You'll come to Fort Lauderdale with me next spring," he said. "You have a beautiful body already. You'll walk down the beach and stop traffic. Trust me."

At the end of the winter, he left for Fort Lauderdale where he spent the early spring months covering the Yankees spring training season. I had three weeks off in March for spring break. I made arrangements with Harry for Annie to stay with him and booked a flight to Florida. I got in to Fort Lauderdale at two o'clock in the morning on a late-night flight made later by delays from an ice storm in New York. Pat was waiting for me at the airport. We walked out into the warm tropical night and the languid breeze that carried the scent of jasmine and the sea. Pat had rented a motel room a block from the ocean. We fell asleep to the rustle of palm fronds outside our window and the faint, soft sound of wind chimes in the sea breeze.

In the morning I unpacked my things. I'd bought a one-piece bathing suit, designed for women who'd had mastectomies, fitted with a special cup for the breast prosthesis. I put the suit on.

"Oh, no," said Pat. "You're not wearing that. Here. Put this on."

He handed me a tiny white string bikini. The top had two triangular patches of white, shiny fabric made to stretch around the breasts with the widest part underneath. The bottom was made of two more little pieces of white material attached to a string that tied around the hips.

"Patty!" I said. "I can't wear that!" I felt my eyes fill with tears.

"Yes, you can," he said. "Just try it on."

I put the tiny bottom on and he stood behind me and slipped the top over my one breast. He tied one pair of strings behind my back and the other around my neck.

"Now hand me your fake boob," he said. He slipped that into the empty pouch of the right side. "Now, take a look at yourself," he said.

He was beaming. I turned to look in the mirror. I looked normally half-naked.

"I guess it's okay," I said. "But what if it falls out?"

"It won't," said Pat. "I've been staring at women with this kind of bathing suit since I got down here. I even went up to one on the beach and asked her if the top ever fell off. She thought I was a pervert. But she told me where to go to find you a bathing suit. It looks fabulous. Let's go get another one."

"Hey, Pat," said the tanned, older woman who waited on us later. "He's been in here every day for the last two weeks staring at bikinis," she said to me. "At first we thought there was something wrong with him, but then he explained what kind of bathing suit he was looking for. And then he told us why. He's very proud of you."

We went down to the beach, to the turquoise sea and the dazzling white sand where the air was heavy with the scent of coconut oil. Men and women lay on the sand, their tanned bodies glistening in the sun. The women all wore a different version of the little string bikini I had on. I looked up at Pat. I saw that he'd been watching me.

"Not one of them has a better body than you do," he said. "I didn't want you to feel different. That bathing suit you brought down would have reminded you of something you lost. I wanted you to see all you've gained."

We spent the days at the beach, in the sun, and the nights at the ballgames. Late at night I lay out on the deck outside of our motel room and stared up at the deep blue tropical sky and the moonlit billowing clouds moving in off the ocean. The warm night wind, rich with the scent of gardenias and jasmine, calmed me, and I was at rest. But every so often I saw a certain sadness cross Pat's face and in those moments he was preoccupied, silent. I knew what troubled him, but I resolved to let him speak of his sadness first.

One night I woke to find myself alone in bed in the darkness. Pat was not in the room. I looked out the window to see him sitting by himself in one of the deck chairs, staring up into the night sky. Then I saw him put his hands up to his face and lean forward, rocking back and forth in the chair. I went out to him. He was crying softly into his hands.

"Patty, what is it?"

"I have to leave her," he said through his tears. "It isn't fair to her . . . the way it is."

"I know."

"I don't know what will happen to my family. It will be very hard."

"What can I do?"

"Try to understand if it takes me awhile to leave. I have to be sure they won't fall apart without me."

"It doesn't matter how long it takes. Isn't there some way we can be together without hurting anyone?"

"I don't know."

"Are we being selfish?"

"Some people will say so."

"Well, that's what they'll say then," I said. "But I won't leave you."

CHAPTER EIGHTEEN

In Stiletto Heels

In the summer of 1981, almost two years after my mastectomy, I decided to get an implant to replace my missing right breast. I went for a routine mammogram before the operation. The x-ray showed some dark spots in the left breast. I went for a second x-ray. Dr. McCullough called me with the results. The shadows were only cysts, but I'd had enough worry.

"I never want to think about cancer again," I said. "I'm too happy to worry. Can you replace the left breast with an implant?"

"Good idea," he said. "We'll put both implants in at once." I made an appointment for the surgery for the first week in July. Annie and Andrew had taken jobs as counselors in a summer camp nearby. Dana had met and married a young sargeant in the Air Force. They were stationed in Germany.

By now Peggy had left the University of Connecticut and rented a house with several of her girlfriends on Fairfield beach. She was thinking of taking some courses at Fairfield University. The train ride from Fairfield into Manhattan was an easy one, less than an hour long, and she was spending much of her time in New York. I thought she might want to come and stay with me for a week or so when I came home from the hospital. I called her. "I'm really happy," I told her. I'm getting two breast implants. Do you think you could come up and stay with me? I haven't seen you and I miss you. And maybe you could help me wash my hair. I won't be able to lift my arms."

"I'm not very good like that, Mom," she said, "and I might have to stay in New York for that week. But I can drive you to the hospital."

She spent the night with me in Wallingford and drove me into New Haven early the next morning. On the way we talked about her plans for the summer and the coming fall. She'd joined the Screen Actors Guild and had already made several national commercials, and she was auditioning for roles in movies and soap operas. She'd changed her name to Meg and chosen my family name, Ryan, as her professional name. Her career was taking off. She wondered if she should move into New York.

"What about college?" I said. "Do you still want to go?" She'd always been an excellent student.

"Yes," she said, "but it's getting harder to get to auditions from Fairfield. Sometimes they want you to be at a place within an hour."

"Well," I said, "you can always go to college. Your career might not wait. What if you do move into New York? Could you go to school there and concentrate on your career at the same time?"

"I'm not sure I can afford to rent there."

"Can you get a roommate?"

"I'll think about it," she said.

We drove up to the hospital entrance. As I got out of the car, she said, "Mom, are you going to be okay?"

"Yes," I said. "I'm not that crazy about hospitals. But this time I'm getting breasts!"

"I love you, Mom."

"I love you, too."

She dropped me at the hospital and then went on to Fairfield to leave the car with Pat so he could drive it back up for me. Pat drove her to the train station. He called me later in my hospital room.

"Are you okay?"

"Yes," I said. "Fine. Why?"

"I asked Peggy how you were on the way to the hospital. She said, 'Oh, you know Mom, she's such a ditz, so twitchy.' I asked her if she understood you and what you went through the last time you were in the hospital. I told her the hospital reminds you of cancer and that you work very hard to get past those memories."

"What did she say when you told her that?"

"Nothing." He paused for a moment, "I don't think your kids are used to anyone sticking up for you."

"I didn't think I was ditzy," I said. "I did tell her I wasn't crazy about hospitals."

"Is she going to stay with you?"

"No," I said. "It's hard to get to New York from Wallingford and she has lots of auditions. She said she's staying in New York for the week."

"I can drive up if you need anything," Pat said. "I'll help you wash your hair."

I came home with my new implants a week later. I couldn't raise my arms, but I felt physically whole again, as if a missing part of my body had been restored. More important, the decision to get them had been all mine.

One afternoon a few days after I got home, I got a phone call from an agent I'd introduced Peggy to, a friend of mine from my days working for the casting director.

"Susan," she said. "This is Shiela. Are you all right?"

"Hi! Yes," I said. "How are you?"

"I'm fine, but we heard that you just came out of the hospital."

"I did," I said. "I just got two gorgeous breast implants!"

"I'm glad everything is all right. We heard you were very ill."

"What?" I said. "I'm not ill. Who said I was?"

"Well, Meg did. She said she needed a few days off from audition-ing to go up to take care of you in Connecticut. Is she there?"

"No," I said. "She isn't. I haven't seen her. I thought she was in New York."

"No, she isn't. When you see her would you have her call me?"

"Yes," I said. "Of course."

I was terrified. Where was she? I called Harry immediately.

"Do you know where she is? Is she all right?"

"She's fine," Harry said. "She's been up on the Cape with Tracy and another friend."

I was absolutely confused. Why did she lie to the agent? Why didn't she want to come and help me if she could? Had I said some-thing to offend her? What? When? I asked Pat.

"Did she say I said anything wrong to her?"

"No."

"Maybe I misunderstood the agent."

"Why would this be your fault, Susan? Why do you always take the blame when one of your kids does something wrong?"

"I'd rather have anything be my fault than theirs."

"Why do you still punish yourself?"

"I guess because I still think I was a bad mother."

In late August, Andrew arrived to begin his junior year at Choate. We moved from the freshman girls' dorm to one of the big old colo-nial houses near the center of the campus, and in September we all started the new school year. Annie and I helped Peggy move into Manhattan. She'd found a roommate and an apartment near New York University, where she wanted to major in journalism. She'd made her dream of living in New York City come true.

I worked out at the gym at school every day of the week, and after a year of exercise, my body was in the best shape it had ever been in. One weekend afternoon when I was working out with Pat at his gym in Fairfield, a young, very large body builder came over to me. He had long blond hair pulled back in a ponytail, and he had on sunglasses with his sweats.

"Excuse me," he said politely. "I wanted to tell you that you have a very hot bod for a mature woman." He ripped his sunglasses off. "Did I say that right? You aren't offended?"

"That is one of the nicest things anyone has ever told me," I said. "Thank you."

In the gym, I was learning the value of setting long-term goals for myself and achieving them, of concentrating only on the future. The men in the gym in Fairfield swore and joked their way through their exercises and laughed to ease the stress of lifting. *If only everyone could laugh their way through stressful moments*, I thought. The men started to include me in their outrageous good humor. I learned to swear like a truck driver. I also learned to think of my body without any embarrassment or shyness. I wore tight jeans, cowboy boots and tight sweaters whenever I went out with Pat. I was proud of myself.

I stopped wearing long, pleated skirts and baggy sweaters to school. Instead, I wore straight, slim skirts with slits up the sides, high heels and silk blouses. Not only had I gained strength and muscle tone in the gym, but I'd also gained self-confidence and assurance. I believed that the weights I lifted in the gym were metaphors for the new power I felt: the heavier the weight, the more strength I had. During a department meeting at the Arts Center I looked around and realized I was the only woman in the theatre department. I was doing the same job as the men; I was a single mother with two children in the school and I was supporting my family all by myself. But I could not overcome the guilt I still felt. Was I a good mother?

The headmaster called me to his office one day and asked me if I'd oversee the two big public relations events at the school: Parents' Weekend, held in October, and Graduation Weekend in June.

"We'd appreciate your help on these two important weekends," he said. "I'd like to introduce you to some of the parents and trustees at a meeting tonight."

At the meeting, he introduced me as "one of our model teachers . . . a strong, smart, independent, single mother." On the way out of the meeting one of the other teachers whispered to me, "He forgot to mention you've got great legs." But all the faculty were "model teachers." The dean of faculty functioned much the way I had as a casting director. He hired the "right" people to fill places according to sex and age within the ranks of teachers. On the Choate campus it was almost as if one was living in a movie. There were equal numbers of young, single teachers and there were young mid thirties married couples with one or two toddlers. There were "middle-aged" teachers in their late forties and fifties, and venerable "older" teachers in their sixties. The year I was hired so was a sixty-two-year-old retired businessman who taught economics, a twenty-one-year-old woman who had just graduated from Radcliffe and would teach English and coach girls' crew, and a young married couple with a one-year-old child. He taught Latin, she taught math and they would live as "houseparents" in one of the dorms. The faculty was as picture-perfect as the place.

As the months went on I realized how much the school counted on the appearance it presented to the outside world. One of the other teachers told me that a former dean had been pressured to leave even though he'd graduated from Choate, as had his father and grandfather before him. He was a handsome, square-jawed man who looked like Tyrone Power. He wore tweeds, smoked a pipe and was accompanied, even into his classroom, by a matching pair of German shepherd dogs. He was the perfect picture of a prep-school dean except that his wife had begun an affair with another woman. The dean's wife ran away with her lover, leaving her husband and their children to face the school community alone. The trustees and administrators of the school politely encouraged him to retire. The school's reputation was more important than the man who had given the best years of his life to it.

The vice principal was a tall, dark woman of French and Armenian descent who spoke four languages, had been educated at Oxford and was always dressed impeccably in the latest French or Italian fashion. At a Christmas cocktail party at her campus residence she introduced me to her husband, a towering black man from Trinidad. He stood a full six-and-one-half-feet tall, and he wore his hair in an upswept, swirling arrangement that added yet another six inches to his height. He had marched with the Black Panthers in New Haven during the anti-Vietnam war riots in the sixties. A teacher, standing near me said, "He was jumping up and down on New Haven Green with Bobby Seale in those days. You couldn't miss him." The vice-principal finished her introduction and left me standing alone with her husband for several minutes. "You're a pretty woman," he said to me in his lilting, Caribbean accent. "Quite a lovely addition to our faculty."

"Thank you," I said and turned away from him.

I felt someone pinch my behind. I turned to look back at the huge man. He smiled and winked at me. Then he turned away. I looked at the teacher standing next to me. "Did you see that?" I said.

"A lot of strange stuff goes on around here," he said. "Appearances aren't everything."

But they seemed to be at Choate. And one of my jobs was to help promote the appearance of the venerable, traditional prep school that was in step with modern times. I was the same age as the wealthy suburban women who came to the school to visit their children for Parents' Weekend. I was the perfect role model, a "mom-away-from-home" to their boys and girls who lived on the sheltered campus. On graduation weekend, I knew how to bring the necessary theatrical flair to the ceremony. Five men wearing tartan kilts and playing bagpipes led the commencement procession across a wide, sun-dappled lawn under tall, old trees. The entire faculty, in full academic regalia, followed the pipers. The graduating class, girls in white dresses and boys in dark suits, followed the faculty.

These ceremonies reassured the parents; the beautiful campus, the handsome faculty and the number of students accepted to Ivy League colleges were all vital to the school's survival. But every so often in the perfect world, an impropriety would occur or a scandal smolder.

At the end of one spring break, three Choate students were arrested at Kennedy airport on their way back to the school from Venezuela where they'd spent the vacation with their families. They were caught with cocaine they were bringing back to the school to sell to other students. The incident made national headlines and news reporters, several from the *New York Times*, made attempts to talk to some of the faculty about the arrests. The headmaster called an emergency meeting of the faculty in the common room of the library. "As you may have noticed," he said, "members of the press and other media have been on campus since yesterday. I'm sure you'll be as polite as always but don't talk to any of them. I don't want this incident blown out of all proportion."

"In proportion to what?" asked a new faculty member, a young recent graduate from Yale. "Three kids got arrested for smuggling drugs. That's pretty serious."

The headmaster couldn't answer. The other new, young teachers in the front row waited expectantly as he searched his mind for an answer. I looked around at the other faculty members. Middle-aged men in frayed tweed jackets and rumpled khaki pants sat in the back rows methodically correcting sheaves of multiple-choice quizzes. Older, unmarried women of the faculty sat in the middle rows, knitting intricately designed sweaters. They all sat without expression, heads bent over the work in their lap.

"I'd like us to hunker down and let this whole thing blow over," the headmaster said, finally.

"Why?" I said.

I saw the headmaster nod at the dean of faculty, an older, shambling man who had himself graduated from the school fifty years earlier. He rose and addressed me.

"Why? Because that's the way we've chosen to do it, Susan. I'm sure you won't have a problem with that. This is the way we've always treated potential scandals around here."

"By sweeping them under the rug, that's how," said one of the older women, not looking up from her knitting. "We've been doing that for as long as I've been here."

"Thank you, lady," said the dean, "for your wry observation."

"It isn't an observation," said the woman. "It is fact." She looked up at him, glowering. "And don't ever call me 'lady' again, mister." She thrust one of her long knitting needles toward him. "I have had my consciousness raised."

The young teacher from the front row raised his hand again.

"If it's true, why don't you want us talking about it?"

The dean of faculty regarded him coldly. "Because the school has a reputation to uphold."

"And don't forget tuitions and future endowments," said another one of the older women. "You have to uphold those, too."

The room went dead silent. The only sound was of the clackety-clack of the knitting needles.

"Thank you," said the headmaster. "That's all."

He adjourned the meeting and asked me and the other teachers who had commented to remain.

"I don't think I have to remind you that some of you have children here at the school and good teaching positions. I'm sure you want to continue so that they can graduate. Certainly you'll want to continue to receive the wonderful benefits this place offers you."

On the way out of the meeting, the vice principal took me aside. "Learn how to cover your ass," she said. "He's trying to do that for the school, and you have to do that for your kids. Say no more."

The incident evoked disturbing memories of my childhood. ("What would people think! Conform or perish!") It was a rude reminder that I was living in an isolated, elite world where the truth could be twisted or hidden to create a desired appearance. I even began to wonder if I'd made the right decision to educate my children here. Was I spoiling them by bringing them to this privileged, unreal place? Would they expect the same privileges when they graduated and went out into the real world? Were they learning that appearance mattered more than the truth?

But I rationalized. Teaching there, I had everything else I wanted for my children. After all, Andrew and Annie lived with me. I could teach them the importance of truth over appearance! The school offered me peace and tranquility and the challenge of my teaching. My two youngest children would be assured of scholarships to good colleges. Dana was in the Air Force, living in Europe and fulfilling her dream of travel. Peggy was fulfilling her dream, too. She was living in New York, auditioning for roles in movies and soap operas. And who knew? Maybe I could even save enough money to buy a house of my own and wait for Pat so we could begin our life together.

In 1982, Pat and his wife separated. He went down to Fort Lauderdale as usual to cover baseball spring training. I flew down for spring break. One Saturday afternoon we were sitting in the sun at the Bootlegger's Lounge pool bar, an outdoor bar on the Intracoastal Waterway. Sailboats and yachts were docked all along the pier next to the pool. The Bootlegger "Hot Bod Bikini Contest" was about to begin. There were eight contestants, young women wearing nothing but stiletto high heels and bikini bathing suits. The string bikinis were made of suede, gold lamé and snake-skin prints. These were never meant to get wet and were designed to wear—as these girls were—with gold jewelry and heavy make-up. Some of the girls were college students, others were young models and some were dancers from the Doll House, Cheetah, the Booby Trap and other nude dance clubs in Fort Lauderdale. The Bootlegger was packed that day with hundreds of tourists and locals, all waiting for the girls, tanned and glistening with oil, to walk around the pool. The girl with the best "hot bod" would receive a seven day, all expenses paid vacation for two in Jamaica, plus $250 spending money.

"You should enter this contest," said Pat. "You have a better body than any of them."

I laughed at him.

"These kids are the same age as my own daughters, Patty."

"So what? You could win this."

"Think so?"

"Why would I lie? I dare you."

"I don't have any shoes."

"Borrow mine," said a young woman sitting next to me. "I think you'd win, too."

I put on the shoes and went over to where the announcer was walking back and forth in front of the judges who were sitting on folding chairs at one end of the pool.

"The world-famous Bootlegger Hot Bod Contest," he bellowed. "Only one rule! Pick the body in the best shape!"

"Can I be a contestant?" I said. "Is there an age limit?"

"You are never too old!" he crowed.

Then he turned to the other contestants.

"Ladies! When I call your name, come out, stand in front of the judges for a minute, walk around the pool, over that little wooden bridge and then back down here in front of the judges. That's all there is to it! Have fun!"

I was the last contestant. He called out my name and as I went out in front of the judges, a roar of applause went up from the crowd. The announcer paused, waiting for quiet.

"You will not believe this, ladies and gentlemen, but this woman is forty-three years old!"

I heard more applause and boat whistles blaring wildly. I was sure it was for the girl who'd gone before me, a platinum blonde with a perfect tan and plump breasts that spilled out of her tiny bikini top. As I walked toward the wooden bridge, a woman my age shouted, "Way to go!" A college boy screamed "All right!" and gave me a thumbs-up sign as I passed him.

I stepped onto the wooden bridge and suddenly realized I had to control my shaking legs. My borrowed stiletto heels were wobbling under my feet like stilts, and I feared I might fall off the bridge, right into the pool. I looked for Pat in the crowd. I saw him jumping up and down, pumping both arms high into the air, shouting, "Yes! Yes!" He grabbed the man standing next to him and began thumping him on the back. I stepped off the bridge and walked around the last side of the pool to face the judges again. They deliberated briefly. I heard the announcer call my name again, and another round of blasts and whistles went off from the boats. The audience began to cheer wildly. In a daze, I realized they were cheering for me. I'd won.

CHAPTER NINETEEN

The New Road

"Cancer is a symbol, as most illness is, of something going wrong in the patient's life, a warning to take another road," wrote Elida Evans. I'd chosen a new road, but I saw that some of the people I loved didn't want to travel with me. My new confidence and strength confused my children. And now that I was learning to live for myself, they seemed to resist me. Their resistance was obvious in small ways.

I came home from the store one afternoon with the car loaded with bags of groceries. I went in and found Andrew lying on the living room sofa, playing his guitar. "Andrew," I said. "Would you help me in with these groceries, please?"

He didn't answer me.

"Andrew," I said. "Didn't you hear me?"

"Yes, Mom. Just a minute. I'm working on this tune."

"Please let that wait. I have things in the car that will melt."

"In a minute."

"No. Now."

He made no move to get up. I went out to the car and started bringing the bags in by myself. Pat drove up. He took several bags out of the car, and we carried them in together. He saw Andrew still lying on the couch, strumming his guitar.

"Andrew," said Pat. "Why aren't you giving your mother a hand with these?"

"Oh, okay," said Andrew, and got up. He started out to the car. "But she's strong," he said over his shoulder. "She lifts all those weights in the gym." He went outside.

Pat looked at me and shook his head.

"You set this up," he said. "You spoiled him. Now he's just behaving like he probably always has."

It was true. I had spoiled him. My children were used to the old "me," the eager-to-please, hungry-for-approval, suburban mom they remembered from their childhood. Now I was becoming someone new, and I felt caught, trapped between that new person I was becoming and the old person they expected me to be. I felt sorry for my children, guilty. I'd taken yet another certitude away from them.

Peggy came up from New York to spend an occasional weekend at Choate. She liked the old traditional campus and the rural setting; it was a respite for her from the city. I felt twinges of guilt that I hadn't been able to give Peggy and Dana the Choate education that I was giving Andrew and Annie. I didn't remind myself that I was doing the best I could for all my children. Instead, I let myself slip into the past and remember the days before I'd left them with their father. If only I had been less confused! If only I'd been stronger! If only I had stayed in the house and their father had left!

Pat drove up one Saturday afternoon to watch a school baseball game while Peggy was there. I put on a T-shirt and a pair of shorts to go with him. I reached up on tip-toe to the top shelf of my closet for my sneakers. I saw Peggy behind me in the closet mirror, staring at my legs. "Mom!" she said. "You're not going out like that, are you?"

"She looks fine," said Pat. He was standing behind her. She hadn't seen him come in. "Your mother's got great legs." I saw a look of annoyance cross Peggy's face. She turned and left the room. I was seeing that the more Pat encouraged me to be myself, the more my children seemed to resent him.

After the game, Pat spent the afternoon making his special spaghetti sauce. Annie and Andrew were going out with friends for the evening. Peggy, Pat and I were alone at dinner. Peggy sat silently poking at the pasta and sauce on her plate. I left the table and went into the kitchen to get some cheese.

"What's the matter, Peg," I heard Pat say. "Don't you like the sauce?"

"It's fine."

"So," said Pat. "I hear you want to be an actress like your mother."

"Do I?"

"Well, you seem to admire her so much, I thought you wanted to be like her."

"Do I?"

"Peg, give me a break. I'm in your corner. I'm not going to come between you and your mother."

"I don't know what you mean," she said, coolly.

I heard her leave the table.

Pat came into the kitchen.

"I don't think she likes you," I said.

"It isn't me," he said. "I don't think she wants anyone to come between you and her."

I wasn't helping the two become better friends. I was torn, guilty that I was spending too much time with him and not enough with her or my other children.

My younger brother came for Easter dinner that year while Pat was in Fairfield. He suggested a walk after dinner. He was fifteen years younger than I, tall and angular, with straight dark hair and our family's light blue eyes. As we walked across the campus he stopped and said suddenly, "You're a scandal. Do you know what people in Fairfield are saying about you?"

"I don't care," I said.

"Pat is a married man with five children."

"Pat is separated from his wife," I said.

"Well, he wasn't for some of the years you've been with him."

"Is any of this your business?"

"Yes. This is a bad reflection on our family. It's a disgrace."

"It's none of your business," I said again.

"Your reputation is in the gutter," he said. "Don't you care?"

"No," I said. "I don't care in the least what you or anyone else thinks."

My brother grew red in the face.

"Whatever happened to you? You used to be so sweet."

"That's it," I said. "You know where your car is." I left him standing there and walked back to my house.

He called after me, "I can't believe you!"

"Why? Because I'm not a pushover anymore?"

"No. Because you're a real bitch now."

"I don't care what you think. It's my life. Go home."

Two months after that episode one of my aunts called me.

"Dear, I've met someone whose son is thinking of enrolling in the school," she said. "Would you be kind enough to show him around the campus? He's an executive with Pepsico, and he's interested in meeting you and seeing the school."

"Sure," I said. "When would he like to come up?"

"Tomorrow," she said.

The man drove up to my house the next morning in a new, dark-blue Mercedes convertible. He was tall and athletic, with close-cropped gray hair and narrow eyes. He wore a white linen shirt, open at the collar, perfectly tailored gray wool slacks and highly polished black loafers with tassels. He had the cool, assured manner of someone used to a great deal of money. Pat arrived at the same time. He wore old jeans and a faded T-shirt. I introduced him to the man and said I'd be back from our tour of the school in an hour.

"Who was that?" said the man as we walked away from my house.

"That's the man I'm going to marry," I said.

"Your aunt didn't say you'd be getting married."

"Why would she?" I said. "Besides, I haven't told anyone in my family."

"Oh?" he said.

"When will your son be coming here to Choate?" I said. "Next fall?"

"My son?" he said. "He's only seven."

I stopped halfway down the driveway. "Well, this tour is silly then, isn't it?"

"Yes," he said. "I guess it is." He looked back up at my house. Pat was sitting on the front porch reading the newspaper. "Nice meeting you," said the man and walked back to his car. I went back to the house and stormed into the kitchen. I dialed my aunt's number.

"What's the matter?" said Pat. "Didn't he like the school?"

"His son is only seven," I said.

"What is he, a child prodigy?" said Pat.

My aunt answered her telephone. "Why did you send that person up here to meet me?" I said. "His son is only in the first grade! How could a little kid be thinking of coming to this school?"

"Now calm down, dear. He's a very nice, divorced man who would like his son to go to a good school. He's quite wealthy." There was annoyance in her tone, but she had acquired a chilly New England charm, that same cool, protective covering that many people in my family used to cover the real emotions they felt. I thought that they were always holding something of themselves back, as if by unleashing any passion they might lose something valuable they would need for future use.

"What does his being wealthy have to do with me?"

"Susan, you're so excitable these days. I was thinking of you, dear. I thought you might like to meet someone who would take good care of you." She paused. "And I don't mean just emotionally."

"Thank you," I said. "But I don't need anyone to take care of me. I'm taking good care of myself." And I hung up.

"What the hell is this with my family?" I said to Pat.

"I don't think they know how to deal with you anymore," he said. "I think they're scared of you."

"Why?"

"They're afraid of what they can't control and they can't control you."

"Good," I said.

In school I was teaching the novels of Edith Wharton. We read *Ethan Frome*, the story of a young man and the stark, cold New England village that smothered his yearnings, killed the bright passion that might have transformed his life, and in the end, destroyed his spirit. We read *The Age of Innocence*, a novel about the doomed love affair between a young scion of an old New York family and a beautiful and exotic countess, their happiness wrecked by the merciless traditions and ferocious expectations of high society and old money, the collective authority of the day.

I thought of the old lessons I was trying to overcome: try to please; nothing is more important than what other people think of you; don't be selfish; think of others first. And I was realizing how difficult it was to rise above the influence of the "collective authority." It requires such strength, as Elida Evans pointed out, "as does not grow overnight."

A senior boy, an anxious, timid student, was struggling along in my class with a C average. He had great difficulty organizing his thoughts on paper, and I was meeting with him twice a week to help him with his essays.

"If you're fearful, you can't think clearly," I said. "What are you scared of?"

"My father really wants me to get into Brown University," he said. "I can't let him down."

"What do you want? We're reading about people who are giving themselves away for others, aren't we?"

"I know, I know. But I want to make him and my mother happy. They've done so much for me. I have to get at least a B in this class!"

"Calm down," I said. "You're a bright kid. Take control of the smallest thing first. Remember what Plutarch said about overcoming little by little. Write one simple sentence at a time. Don't worry about failing."

"Okay," he said.

I had assigned a long essay that would count for a third of the final exam grade. It was on any topic of the students' choice and due on the last day of class. The boy plagiarized the long essay. I had to notify the dean, who called the boy's father. The man rushed to the school and met with me in my office.

"He tries so hard," he said. "Can't you raise the grade at all?"

"I'm trying to make sure he isn't expelled," I said. "In his favor, he admitted taking another student's work. He's sorry, and he's very upset, but I can't give him a higher grade."

The man reached into the inside breast pocket of his suit coat and took out his wallet.

"Can I make any contribution to you or the school?"

"Absolutely not," I said.

"I'm sorry," he said and put his wallet away. "What should I do?" asked the man. "We're spending all this money to give him a good start."

"Tell him to relax," I said. "I don't think anything in life is more important than peace of mind, and your son doesn't have that. He's too anxious to please, and he has no idea what he wants for himself. That's scary. Your son is scared."

"Well, life is tough," he said. "He'd better get used to the pressure."

"Excuse me, but I think life is easier when you aren't scared. You can think better."

"How would you know that?" he said.

"It's a long story."

The boy graduated with his class, but he wasn't accepted into Brown. He came to see me at home before he left Choate.

"Thanks for sticking up for me," he said. "I really didn't want to go to Brown to begin with."

"You could have said so," I said. "You can stick up for yourself, you know." Then I asked, "Did you cheat on purpose?"

He didn't answer me.

I went upstairs to Annie's bedroom and sat down on her bed. She was sitting at her desk doing her homework. "Do I put pressure on you to do well here?" I said.

"Of course not, Mom. I like the work. But I think some kids feel over their heads here, and they can't tell anyone."

"But you would tell me if I pressured you?"

"Mom! I said you weren't! Why do you worry so much about what we think?"

Why? Because my children were my "collective authority." I was still overcome by my feelings of failure and guilt about having left them. I was still under their influence, still trying to gain their approval. I was tough and confident with my students in my classes. I was myself with everyone else's children—but not my own.

CHAPTER TWENTY

Into the Wind

Trying to overcome the guilt I felt about my children was like beating into the wind. It seemed that I was like a small boat trying to make even a little headway, but always losing more than I gained. I was troubled always by the thought that as I was making myself stronger, I was hurting my children. I was leaving them again. They wanted their old mother back, but that woman was gone forever. A new woman was in her place, a woman they either didn't understand or didn't want to understand. I tried to remember my grandmother's words of so many years ago, "What's done is done. You must look ahead."

Peggy had won her first movie role, playing Candice Bergen's daughter in the film *Rich and Famous*. She invited me to the premiere in New York. I told Pat I was going in to meet her in the city.

"Oh!" he said. "I've never been to a premiere. Can I come along?"

"Oh, no," I said. "I don't think she wants you to come. I think she just wants me to be there with her."

"Is that what she said?"

"No, but I'm sure that's what she wants."

"How do you know?" he snapped. He was hurt and angry. "Did you ask her if I could come along?"

"No."

"You're afraid to upset her."

"It's not that," I said. "I don't think she likes you."

"It's not me. She doesn't even know me. All she sees is that I'm someone who might come between you and her."

"I understand that! I left her! She thinks it's happening again!"

"Is that why you're not afraid of pissing me off, but you're terrified of annoying her?"

"This is her big night. I don't want to hurt her!"

"You're hurting her by not giving her the chance to say yes or no!" He was furious with me. "No wonder your kids don't understand you. You're never straight with them! You are strong with everyone but them."

I went alone with Peggy to her premiere. I was afraid of upsetting her.

Andrew graduated from Choate in 1982 and won a full academic scholarship to Tulane University. He came home for Thanksgiving vacation. Over the weekend, one of his friends invited him to a party, but he hadn't brought any dress shirts back with him and he needed one.

"Why didn't you bring one back with you?" I said.

"I lost them, Ma. I do my own laundry, and I just don't know what happened to them."

"Andrew, you've been losing your things for years."

"What things?"

"Remember all those bicycles? Try to keep track of your stuff. I really can't afford to keep replacing your dress shirts."

"Who said you had to keep replacing all of them? I just asked if you could buy me one."

"No."

"Why?"

"I can't afford it. Borrow one."

"Why can't you afford it? Probably because you spend all your money going down to see Pat."

"Mind your own business, Andrew. Or better yet, get a part-time job. That way if you lose a shirt it's your problem and not mine."

"Think of yourself, Mom. That's typical."

"Andrew, I'm sitting here doing schoolwork. I'm trying to support us. You're interrupting me."

I didn't buy the dress shirt, and Andrew refused to talk to me for the rest of the vacation. He returned to school. I felt horrible. After all, he was away at college, away from home for the first time. Maybe it was hard for him to concentrate on his laundry and his grades at the same time. How could I be so hard on him? How could I expect him to get a part-time job? I didn't hear from him again until he called me right before he was due to come home at Christmas.

"Ma! I got a great job!"

"Where?"

"I'm a part-time waiter at Arnoud's! It's a beautiful restaurant in the French Quarter!" He sounded thrilled.

"That's wonderful Andrew!"

"Mom, I know you'll probably be upset, but I lost my dress shoes and the manager says I can't wear my sneakers to work. I really need a pair right away."

"How much do you need? I'll send the money right away."

"Thanks, Ma."

"Can you get home for Christmas?"

"Yeah! Can't wait to get home. I want to talk to you about something, too." Toward the end of the vacation he came into the living room where I sat reading.

"I've decided not to go back to school," he said. He didn't look at me, but sat down on the sofa and began to lace up his sneakers.

"What?! Why?"

"I don't like New Orleans. I don't like the school. Besides, all the kids I know have so much money, and I can't afford to do anything but just go to school. I can't afford to even go out."

"But you have a full four-year scholarship!"

"I know, Ma. But I just don't want to go back."

I tried to organize my thoughts. Did he want the security of home? I remembered what I was like at eighteen when I'd fled college in Boston, when I was childlike, self-absorbed, confused by my liberty, when I'd needed the security of other people telling me what to do. Were these the reasons Andrew wanted to leave college?

"Andrew, when I was your age, I went away to college. But then I quit and went home after two semesters. I was confused and scared. I should have had the courage to stay and figure out how to be a stronger person, to get by on my own, but I didn't. My parents let me come home. I wish they hadn't."

"What are you telling me? That I can't?"

"I'm telling you what I think your options are. You can leave Tulane, come back to Connecticut and get a job and your own apartment. Or, you can get a part-time job, your own apartment and go to some local college at night. Or you can go into the service. Or you can stay at Tulane. Living here at home is not one of your options. I have one last question. Why did you need money for dress shoes if you weren't planning to go back to school and your job?"

He didn't answer. Instead he stood up and hurled his sneakers against the wall.

"I'm not going back! You can't make me! I'll do what I want!"

He grabbed his sneakers, stormed out the front door and slammed it violently behind him. Snow was falling heavily outside. He had left without his coat. Annie rushed down the stairs into the living room.

"Mom! What happened?"

"Andrew doesn't want to go back to Tulane. He wants to come back and live at home, and I told him he couldn't. I told him he had to be strong enough to start living on his own."

Annie started to cry.

"How can you be so hard on him, Mom? You never listen to us anymore! Can't we ever have a normal family? Nothing has ever been right since you left!"

"Annie, nothing remains the same!" I said.

She fled back upstairs to her room. I waited for hours for Andrew to come home. At nightfall the phone rang. It was the mother of one of his friends in Wallingford.

"Andrew is here," she said. "I thought you'd like to know."

"Thank you, " I said. "May I talk to him, please?"

Andrew came on the phone.

"Andrew," I said. "Please come home."

"No," he said. "You don't want me."

On the day Andrew was to return to school, I called his friend who was driving back down to New Orleans. I gave the friend Andrew's suitcase and told him where he was staying. But Andrew wouldn't go back to school. Instead he stayed with another friend in Wallingford for the next three months. He refused to see me or talk to me. I was determined to be strong, but I agonized. Had his privileged Choate education insulated him from the realities of the "outside" world? Had I spoiled him and then insisted that he go out on his own? Was I being fair? I fought with myself mightily, caught again between the storm of my feelings and the calm of clear thoughts. But somehow I held firm.

And so I continued on with my children, in erratic fits and starts, never on an even keel, overreacting and underreacting, always battling with myself, always haunted by the fear that they would think I didn't love them enough. No sooner would I overcome one guilt feeling than I had to turn around and overcome another one from a different direction. I remembered the lifeguard who, so many years before, had taught me to sail.

"Tighten your sail and take the rudder with a firm hand. Don't give up. If you let out too much sail and lose your grip, the wind will blow you over. You'll capsize and go down."

Somehow I knew that the smallest weakness would be a betrayal of myself and my health. Those small betrayals might accumulate, and I might lose the self-control I'd finally gained. I was learning to live within, to become, finally, an individual strong enough to overcome losses and disappointments. My mother and my grandfathers had succumbed to that downward spiral of fear, helplessness and loss of self. I'd fought against that spiral and came out alive. Now I had to fight another battle. I would not allow guilt to have power over me. I would not live for others. I wouldn't live to please. I had to live for myself. I wouldn't capsize. I wouldn't go down. I struggled on.

When Annie graduated from Choate in 1984, I resigned my position there. The school had been a saving place for me. It had provided peace and security so I could begin my new life and provide for my children. The school gave me everything I needed then—even sent someone to rake leaves in fall and shovel the snow from my walk in winter. But the big, old colonial house where we lived wasn't mine. Like the apartments in which I'd lived in New York, it belonged to someone else, to the school. There was a price for the security and comfort the school offered. It was necessary to conform to all the traditions, to "fit in," to look the other way when something "improper" occurred that might threaten the school's reputation. The beautiful world of Choate reminded me of the traditional town of my childhood. It was safe but closed. And I was changed. I'd changed myself, found the independent girl I'd once been. I was in control of my own life. It was time to go out into the real world.

Pat and I moved to Fort Lauderdale the autumn after I left Choate. I'd never forgotten the warmth and the ease of the weeks I'd spent in Fort Lauderdale. I always thought of it as the place where my new life had begun. We were married quietly at sunset on Christmas Eve in 1984 on the deck of our small apartment overlooking the Intra-coastal Waterway.

Annie was my bridesmaid. Palm trees stood in dark silhouettes against a pink and crimson sky. A clutch of sailboats rocked gently at their moorings around the dock below us. Their tall masts, strung with tiny white lights, swayed in the deepening twilight. I heard the sound of a softly clanging ship's bell and the laughter of our friends and the tinkle of ice in glasses. I saw Pat standing with a group of our guests. I watched him throw back his head and laugh with them. I saw him look for me and then, as he caught my eye, I saw him smile at me. He came over to me and put his arm around me and hugged me to him. We stood together for a moment and looked across the waterway, out to the ocean beyond. We watched the great, high white clouds sailing across the tropic night sky like huge sailing ships, full of beauty and possibility. I remembered the single rose and the card he'd left me in the hospital years before. I remembered the words he had written. "Hurry! We have a life to live." My life with him was just beginning.

CHAPTER TWENTY-ONE

In Hollywood

My life with my children was changing. Slowly, they were getting to know the new "me," and I was growing more relaxed with them, closer to them and more confident in my relationships with them. Andrew returned to Tulane. He'd almost lost his scholarship, but he talked to his dean and his teachers and he spent several summers taking courses to make up for the ones he'd missed. He was a gifted student and a talented songwriter and singer. When he graduated from Tulane in 1986, he stayed on in New Orleans waiting for Annie to graduate from Adelphi in New York. She had a beautiful voice, bright, clear and powerful, and Andrew was hoping to form a songwriting and singing partnership with her.

He came often to visit us in Fort Lauderdale, and on those visits I noticed that he was restless, anxious. I knew he moved frequently in New Orleans, from apartment to apartment. On one visit I said, "If you're flying around all the time, you can't make a nest. You might feel calmer when you have your own place." He sent me a card after he went back to New Orleans. "It's hard to thank you for everything you do for me. It makes me proud to see you so smiling and alive. I know I have a tough time showing it, but you should always know how much love I have for you."

Annie was ready to start her last year in college when she decided to have some surgery done on her foot that she'd put off. I flew up to be with her while she was in the hospital on Long Island. Pat flew up on the day she was released, and the three of us drove into New York, where he had meetings with several magazine editors. We planned to stay overnight in the city, them fly back with Annie to Fort Lauderdale where she could relax in the sun for several weeks before starting school. Pat booked a suite of rooms in a grand, old hotel on Park Avenue.

"Swell," said Annie as we drove up to the entrance.

A uniformed doorman helped her out of the car, and handed her crutches to her and helped her up marble steps into the lobby. She sank into a deep, plush chair in the lobby while Pat registered us at the hotel desk. Upstairs, she and I settled in while Pat went off to his meetings.

"What would you like?" I said.

"Aaah," she said. "I'd like a hot bath. That hospital smelled."

I drew a bath in the deep, old-fashioned porcelain tub. She got in and draped her bandaged foot over the edge of the tub to keep it dry. "Now what would you like?" I said.

"Room service," she said.

She sat in the hot tub, ate a chicken salad and sipped a glass of chilled, white wine.

"Oh, boy," she said. "Ain't this the life?"

She was learning to put some of her needs first. I was happy for her. In Fort Lauderdale, she wrapped a giant white sock over her bandaged foot and walked with a cane down to the beach. She sat and read and dozed in the sun for two weeks before she went back to New York to finish her last year of school.

I flew out to California to visit Dana and her new husband, who were stationed near Sacramento; Pat and I flew to New Orleans several times to visit Andrew; and Annie spent her long school vacations with us in Fort Lauderdale. Peggy was the only distant child.

She'd spent two years on the soap opera, *As the World Turns*, and in 1984 she decided to leave the show and move from New York out to Los Angeles. One night, very late, the phone rang. Peggy was calling from California. She was in tears. Her beloved acting teacher had died suddenly.

"Mom, I just thought how awful it would be if anything happened to you before I could tell you I love you."

"I love you, too, Peg," I said. "Don't worry. Nothing's going to happen to me. Everything's fine."

She called me often after that night. Sometimes, later at night, she reached Pat after I'd fallen asleep. She confided in him. She was concerned about her career. She'd made another movie since *Rich and Famous*, but most of the work she'd done had been in television in New York. Now that she'd moved out to Los Angeles her movie career seemed stalled, and she was frightened. The only thing she'd been offered was the role of a ditzy blonde college student in a sitcom starring Lisa Bonet, and she was thinking of taking it.

"If you take it, you'll never be an actress," Pat told her. "You'll just be stereotyped as a dumb, ditzy blonde. If you want the money, take the part. But if you really want to be an actress turn it down and keep plugging away." She turned the sitcom down and auditioned for a role in a movie with John Candy and Eugene Levy, called *Armed and Dangerous*. She won the role, and although the movie was panned, *People* magazine called her "an unexpected pleasure . . . Meg Ryan is an up-and-comer." She was thrilled but still anxious. Pat considered her confidences with great care. He began to feel close to her. I was worried about her, and I missed her. I told Pat, "She's all by herself out there, and she's scared."

"I'm going out on a story next month," he said. "You'll come with me and see her." Before we could leave she called us. She'd started filming a movie with Tom Cruise and Anthony Edwards called *Top Gun*. She had a small role as the wife of Anthony Edwards, another promising young actor, and she'd be busy for several months. Could we come out when the filming was over? In the winter of 1985, months before *Top Gun* was released, Pat was assigned a story in San Diego, and I flew out to California with him. We planned to drive up to Los Angeles and stay with Peggy for one night before going home to Florida.

She was spending much of her time with Tony Edwards at his house in the Hollywood Hills, but she'd rented an apartment on Venice Beach and she insisted we stay there. We had dinner with her in Santa Monica, dropped her at Tony's house, and then drove to Venice Beach. The neighborhood was rundown and seedy. Dopers sat on the street corners, staring furtively at cars, and the streets smelled of urine. Peggy's apartment was a dingy, one-room studio overlooking an alley several blocks back from the beach. It didn't look like a place she spent much time in—sparsely furnished, no plants, no photos, nothing that looked as if it belonged to her. Police sirens sounded all night long, and we heard drunken voices in the alley below arguing and screaming at each other. We hardly slept. "This is horrible," I said to Pat. "I have to tell her." We left the place at six in the morning and drove to the airport where I found a phone and woke her at Tony's house.

"Peg," I said. "I don't want to tell you what to do, but your apartment's in an awful neighborhood. I worry that you won't be safe there. Can you move from there?"

"Thanks, Mom," she said. "But don't worry. I'm thinking of

finding another place with a roommate. For now I'll stay with Tony."

Top Gun opened in Fort Lauderdale in the summer of 1986. Pat and I went to see it the night it opened. I remember being very nervous as the opening credits came onto the screen. Like all mothers, I wanted my child to be wonderful in the movie and for the audience to love her for her sake. Most of all, I wanted her to have her dream.

In the movie, she played the wife of a young fighter pilot who is killed on a training mission. In one of the last scenes in the movie, she is sitting in a darkened room, mourning her lost husband, when Tom Cruise comes into the room to find her. He sits down next to her to share her sorrow. The sight of Peggy's tear-stained face on a movie screen, larger than life, was heartbreaking to me. The audience was looking at her as an actress playing a character, but I was only able to see my daughter and her anguish seemed too real to me, too much. I wanted to stop the projector and call out, "Stop! Don't cry, Peg! It's only a movie! It's make-believe!"

Several months later, she and Tony flew to Fort Lauderdale and spent several days with us. I was relieved to see how confident and happy she was. She was a young hard-working, promising actress whose career was just beginning.

The day they left, I drove them to the airport. Just before she boarded her plane she kissed me good-bye. "I'm glad you're so happy, Mom. I'm proud of you in your new life," she whispered. She smiled at me, and I saw my daughter again as she had been, the infant gazing up at me with her trusting, translucent eyes, the little girl who leaped with blonde hair flying into my arms from the school bus, the eager, happy girl she'd been until that terrible day when she was fifteen and those pale blue eyes were filled with tears and anguish. Tears filled my own eyes. "I'm sorry it's taken so long for us to be this close again," I said. "Let's never be far apart again."

"You're my mother, and I love you," she said. "How could we be far apart?" She smiled again and then turned and walked down the narrow jetway to board her plane. At the end she stopped and looked back at me. She smiled once more and waved. She blew me a kiss, turned the corner and was gone.

A short time after that trip, she broke off her relationship with Tony. She'd met the actor Dennis Quaid while filming the movie *Innerspace* in 1987 and made a second movie with him called *D.O.A.* She called me from the movie set. "Mom, I think I have a love crush on Dennis!"

"Which is it?" I asked. "Love? Or a crush?!"

"Love! He is so incredibly sweet!" She seemed ecstatic. I was thrilled for her.

They came to Fort Lauderdale for a short visit with us in late summer of 1988. Dennis was a tall, raw-boned Texan, thin and wiry, and full of a kind of jittery nervous energy. They were obviously smitten with each other, and I remember being surprised to hear him call her Meg. I realized that my daughter had a life of her own, one that I knew little about and this was as it should be. She was on her own, making her own way, in charge of herself and her career. I was delighted for her.

She'd brought a script with her called *When Harry Met Sally*, and she was very excited about filming the movie. She sat down in the kitchen and read parts of the role of Sally Albright to me as I made dinner. The movie was a romantic comedy, about two old friends who discover that they can be lovers and friends. When it was released my daughter was no longer an "up-and-comer." She would now be a famous movie star.

I didn't see her until the end of that year. She called to invite us to a New Year's Eve party at Dennis's house in L.A. We flew out, arrived in Los Angeles at nine on New Year's Eve and drove to Dennis's house on a hill overlooking Hollywood. Peggy met us at the door. I was shocked to see how tired and thin she looked. The healthy glow that had always been hers was gone, and her face looked sallow and drained. "Are you all right?" It was the first question I asked her.

"I'm fine, Mom." She looked impatient, as if my question irritated her. I wondered if she were just overtired.

Inside, the kitchen was crowded with young actors and actresses, several of whom I recognized, all dressed in black, leaning insouciantly against the counters or slouched in chairs. The kitchen table and counters were littered with paper plates, leftover food and half-empty bottles of expensive champagne. I saw the actor Keifer Sutherland, who had appeared with Peggy in a small movie called *Promised Land*, sitting in a kitchen chair looking tired, small and watchful. No one seemed to have much to say except for an occasional comment about a script, or a movie or a part.

Suddenly Dennis burst into the kitchen. The guests in the kitchen watched him as he rushed about, opening cabinets and pouring more spices into a large pot of gumbo that simmered on the stove. Suddenly he spotted us. "Well, hey, Meg's mom! Pat!" He hugged me and put his arm around Pat.

"What'll you have, Pat?"

"Bourbon and water, if you have it."

"Sure," he said. "I'll have one, too. How 'bout you, Kiefer? Want a drink?"

"I'll make my own," said the actor. "I take my bourbon straight." Dennis handed Pat his drink. "You know, Meg told me you were a professional baseball player," he said. "I was a boxer, you know."

"Really," said Pat. "I didn't know that."

"Well, yes I was."

He seemed anxious with Pat, deferential, as if trying to impress Pat with some sports expertise of his own. He turned and smiled at me. He had a coy, flirtatious smile and a kind of cocky assurance with me that he didn't have with Pat.

"You're so pretty! You look like your daughter!"

"It's the other way around, Dennis," said Pat.

"Oh? Yeah!"

Peggy and I went out into the living room. More paper plates and empty plastic glasses littered the floor. Overflowing ashtrays sat on tables that were wet with spilled drinks. On the mantel was a framed, recent cover of G.Q. magazine with Dennis's picture on it. Someone had scrawled across the bottom, "Dennis Quaid lies to G.Q."

Groups of young people sat around the room talking quietly among themselves. They seemed lifeless somehow, almost as if they'd relied on the films they were in to give them energy they didn't have.

A woman with red hair sat alone on the sofa in the middle of the room, smoking a cigarette. She wore long black leggings that were faded and stained and a baggy black sweater. Peggy introduced her as Bonnie Raitt, the singer. I sat down next to her.

"I'm happy to meet you," I said. "I remember your father in *Carousel* on Broadway." The woman looked at me blankly.

"Your father is John Raitt, right?" She nodded. "I had a big crush on him when I was a girl," I said.

She smiled vaguely. She was about to reply when Dennis rushed into the living room. He yanked the piano bench out from under a baby grand piano and sat down.

"This is from my new movie!" he announced.

He began to pound on the keys of the piano and sing "Goodness, gracious, great balls of fire!" in a pale but loud imitation of Jerry Lee Lewis.

"He's my idol!" he shouted.

Then he got up and raced out of the room. I looked at the woman sitting next to me. She lit another cigarette and stared absently after Dennis. I looked at the other silent actors and actresses gathered around the room. I wondered, *Were they as flat and one-dimensional as they seemed, or was I expecting more?* They seemed larger than life on the movie screen, but had the screen magnified them, given them a depth they really didn't have? And were they lazy now, expecting celluloid to give them life and color?

I couldn't think of anything else to say. I excused myself and went to find Pat. I went toward the back of the house, down a small hallway, past the open door of a bedroom. I caught a glimpse of Dennis sitting by himself on the bed, staring, dully, straight ahead, at nothing. He looked spent, as if his efforts to entertain had exhausted him. I found Pat outside on a back deck, smoking his cigar.

"I'm either too old or too tired," I said. "But it's a real effort to get anyone to talk here. No one speaks!"

"I know," said Pat. "Maybe we just don't know enough about movies."

I went in to look for Peggy. Now Dennis was back in the kitchen, perched on a kitchen counter, playing his guitar and singing a song he'd written. Peggy was moving between people, silently gathering up the stacks of dirty paper plates and plastic glasses.

"Can I help you?" I said.

"No, that's okay," she said.

She looked exhausted. She glanced over at Dennis who was still singing.

"I'm really tired. I'll go to bed before he will."

"I think we'll go to bed early, too," I said. "Both of us are tired from the flight."

"Okay, Mom," she said. "Goodnight."

Shortly after that New Year's Eve party, I flew out to Los Angeles again with Pat on one of his assignments. Peggy and I had lunch with her manager and another friend. Peggy wore lace-up black boots and a long, baggy black jumper with a white T-shirt underneath. She was even thinner than when I'd last seen her several months before. Her manager and the friend both wore dark business suits with short skirts and silk blouses. I wore a black leather mini-skirt, black stockings, high heels and a sweater.

"Wow!" said Peggy's manager. "You don't look at all like I expected!"

"What did you expect?" I said, laughing.

The manager looked at Peggy and then seemed uneasy, at a loss for words. "Well," she said, "Meg said you had . . ."

"Oh," I said. "Breast cancer. Yes. I did years ago."

"She never said you were in such great shape!" She stopped, flustered. "I mean you look wonderful!" She looked at Peggy again. "Meg! Your mother looks so much like you! So, ah, so L.A.! She looks like, ah . . . like . . ." She couldn't seem to find words to finish her sentence.

"I look like me," I said. "I dress this way because I want to." The woman still looked confused. I tried to explain. "This isn't L.A.," I said. "This is me. The real me."

After lunch Peggy and I drove up to Santa Barbara to keep an appointment she'd made there with a real estate agent. She wasn't sure that she wanted to stay in Los Angeles.

"I don't think I want to live so close to Hollywood," she said.

"I don't blame you," I said. I told her a story I'd once heard about Rosalind Russell at a Hollywood party. She was in the ladies room, in one of the stalls, when she overheard several women talking about her. They didn't know she was there. "Roz is in Hollywood, but she's not of Hollywood," they said. The actress waited until the women left and then rushed out to find her husband. She told him what the women had said. "My feelings are so hurt!" she cried. "Why?" asked her husband. "That's a compliment. It means you work here, but you're not part of the whole sideshow."

"Hmmm," Peggy said. "Do you think it's a sideshow?"

"I don't know if it's a sideshow," I said. "But it doesn't seem real. Your manager didn't seem to understand me when I tried to explain myself. I couldn't live in a world where people don't understand what 'real' means."

"Hmmm," she said again. I had the feeling I was talking too much. But did she understand what I meant?

On the way back from Santa Barbara, she said, "Mom, I want you to tell me what you think of Dennis."

"Well," I began, "he's a very sweet man and . . ." I stopped myself. "Do you want me to tell you what I think, or what you want to hear?" She looked over at me, surprised.

"Mom . . . tell the truth."

"He seems child-like. Undisciplined." I paused for a minute, remembering the guests at his New Year's Eve party. "But maybe that's Hollywood. Maybe it's difficult to get to know the real person under what appears to be real." I looked over at her, waiting for her to answer. She stared ahead at the road and said nothing.

That night we made plans to meet at the Ivy, one of Peggy's favorite restaurants in Santa Monica. She asked me to call the manager and make the reservations.

"They know me there. Just say you're my mother and that I asked you to call."

I called the manager. "My daughter asked me to call and make reservations for three," I said.

"Who's your daughter?"

"Meg Ryan."

The manager laughed. "Right," he said. "I get a lot of calls from people who use stars' names to get in here."

I was mortified. "No!" I said. "She asked me to call!"

"Have her call," he said and hung up. I called Peggy to tell her what had happened but there was no answer. We went to the Ivy anyway and waited outside for Peggy. We waited for a half-hour. Finally Pat went to the manager and asked if Peggy was in the restaurant. The manager was annoyed. "Somebody else called here trying to get in," he said.

"Yes," Pat said. "Her mother called. We were supposed to meet her here for dinner."

"Meg Ryan isn't here and we have no tables," the manager said.

We drove back to our hotel, and I tried Peggy again. She picked up the phone.

"Where were you?" I said.

"Oh! Something came up, Mom. I tried to get you, but you weren't in your room."

"We were at the restaurant! Why didn't you call there?" I told her what the manager had said. "People try to use stars' names to get in that restaurant."

"Hmmm," she said. "Well, I'm really sorry, Mom. Look, I have to go. I'll see you in the morning."

I was confused and embarrassed. I told Pat. "Why would she do that?" I asked.

"It's almost as if she was setting you up to look foolish," he said.

"I don't understand," I said.

Peggy was filming the movie *Presidio* with Sean Connery and Mark Harmon. She wanted to introduce me to her two co-stars. Mark Harmon was a very handsome and courteous young man who insisted on showing me a family album he'd brought along to the set. Sean Connery was resting in his trailer.

"Peg, he's resting," I said. "I can meet him some other time."

"Mom!" she said. "He'd love to meet you."

"Really, Peg. Another time."

"It'll just take a minute!"

She took my hand and pulled me toward his trailer. Peggy knocked on the door. There was no answer.

"Peg, please!"

She knocked on the door again, more sharply. I was mortified. The door opened and there stood the actor, handsome as ever, but in his bathrobe. He had obviously been napping.

"Sean!" said Peggy. "This is my mom."

"Hello," he said in his gruff, Scottish brogue. "Please, come in."

"Oh, no," I said. "You were resting."

"Please," he said. "I insist." There was nothing to do but go in.

"My husband is a great fan of yours," I said. "And so am I. It really is a pleasure to meet you."

He grinned broadly. "Well, I'm glad I'm liked," he said. "But I'm afraid today is not one of my best. I've got a headache and my head feels as big as a biscuit tin."

"I hope you'll feel better," I said. "It was wonderful to meet you."

"My pleasure," he said and kissed my hand.

As we walked away from his trailer, Peggy said, "I just thought you'd love to meet him, Mom. You've always liked him."

"Yes," I said. "But I wish we hadn't disturbed him."

"He wasn't disturbed! He's a huge star!"

Months later, just before the movie opened, Pat and I were laying in bed watching *Entertainment Tonight* on television. Peggy was being interviewed. She told the interviewer a funny story about Sean Connery and the day she brought her mother to the set of the movie.

"My mother was such a ditz!" Peggy said, giggling and tossing her head. "She practically beat down his trailer door to get at him!"

I sat up in bed and blurted out at the television. "That wasn't the way it happened!"

"What?" Pat said.

"That wasn't it at all!"

"What the hell are you talking about?"

I told him. "I guess she needed a cute story about her ditzy mother to sell some tickets," he said.

"But that's not the way it happened! It isn't true!"

As Peggy's career was burgeoning, I began to read about myself in the interviews she gave to magazines. In some of the articles she referred to me as her "much-admired, schoolteacher mother, who first encouraged her to become an actress." In others she said I was a "part-time casting director" who had helped her to get her first movie role. She never mentioned my stage-acting experience when she talked about me to interviewers. I wondered why she left that fact out.

In those early interviews, she referred to herself as a student "one semester short of getting a degree in journalism" and to her blossoming career as having "happened by accident." She presented herself as a young woman who had weathered her parents' divorce and come through the experience as a stronger person. "She seems grounded, solid," wrote one reporter. Pat brought home a copy of *Rolling Stone* magazine later that year.

"Read what your daughter said about you," he told me. "She said a terrific thing."

I looked at the sentence he pointed out. "What she [Meg] learned from her much admired mother, she says, is making sure you're responsible for yourself . . . an independent soul who comes to someone else, whole." I let out a long sigh. "Finally," I said. "Maybe my children will all understand what I've been trying to show them."

I'd hoped that by becoming an individual myself I was showing my children the strengths they could gain. I wanted them to know how important it is to be free of what other people think, to be free of guilt. The truth was that I had vowed never to let people have power over me again—including my own children.

CHAPTER TWENTY-TWO

An Existential Shift

Self-healers are all the same.
The results they achieve are
no coincidence.

BERNIE SIEGEL
PEACE, LOVE AND HEALING

In Florida, I volunteered for the American Cancer Society's "Reach to Recovery" program. Members of the program, women who have overcome breast cancer, visit those women in the hospital who have just had mastectomies. I felt a tremendous bond with these women I went to see, a great responsibility to them to share my health if I could. I forced myself to go into the area hospitals. I made myself remember how frightened I was on the day of my mastectomy. I wanted to give these women the care that I'd received, calm their fears and give them hope. I'd healed myself and recovered my health and my will to live. I wanted them to see that they could, too.

The rule for the volunteer was to listen and to share personal experiences only when asked. So I didn't talk. I listened. For most of the women I met, it was enough for them just to see me standing in front of them years after I'd overcome the illness they were facing. The first place the women looked was at my bosom so I always wore a tight sweater. The first question most of them asked was how I stayed in such good shape. "At the gym," I'd say. "An hour a day. I'm in charge of my body." They'd look at me and nod. Then they would begin to talk.

Their experiences were almost all the same. Each seemed to be like the kind of person I had been; they were extraverted women, people pleasers, who had been living for others. They'd suffered a severe, intensely personal emotional trauma, always a loss of some kind, a private loss that was unknown to friends or family because they felt unable to communicate their sorrows. The loss was of someone or something that they'd been living for, and it had occurred in the six to eighteen months preceding the onset of the disease. The loss for these women with breast cancer was almost always related to children or husband; many, like myself, had recently been divorced. They believed they had failed to nurture those closest to them. They felt unable to cope not only with the event, but with any part of their lives. They told me that they felt physically and emotionally exhausted just before the onset of the illness and that this was a certain kind of exhaustion, a fatigue of the mind and the muscles. There was an ache behind the eyes. Sometimes the effort to keep their eyes open was too much. Nothing could ease the tiredness and sleep would not come. Right before the cancer struck, there was an overwhelming feeling of helplessness, then hopelessness, then despair. I found it uncanny, mysterious, that their stories were almost all the same and so like mine.

There were several amazing details. The women were, as I had been, terrified that cancer would strike them in the very part of the body it eventually did. They were enduring a kind of strange, self-fulfilling prophecy; they had half-expected the very disease they were dreading. I remembered that my worst fear had been of breast cancer. I had thought that would be the way I would die. I believed that the loss of my breast would be a punishment for my failure as a mother, daughter and wife.

The women had had nightmares, strange and grotesque dreams that they couldn't understand, in the months preceding the illness. I remembered those terrible nights in the strange apartments in New York and the dreams I had had of mute women cut in half, sliced, neatly down the middle, empty women with empty eyes, dressed as mimes, performing for others . . . women who were without breasts. I remembered what Elida Evans had written about the dreams people have that often symbolize their cancers before they are even diagnosed. "The dream is always a message to the sleeper," she wrote. The women in my dream were symbols of myself separated from myself, lost, mute and without a breast.

I was curious to know why cancer begins, as Evans also questioned, "in one place and not all over the body." She theorized that cancer strikes in that part of the body that is most closely associated with the emotional loss or trauma. "In women it is most frequently the maternal organs, as though there had been in the patient an unsatisfied maternity . . . as the breast is visible and considered beautiful evidence of motherhood, it is even more the seat of motherhood than the uterus." No wonder the cancer had struck me in the very physical symbol of motherhood and femininity. The loss of my breast seemed to represent the losses I believed I'd caused as a mother and daughter and wife.

I thought of a distant cousin of mine, a quiet, scholarly man in his late forties who'd never married. He went to Thailand to research a doctoral dissertation and fell in love with a young Thai girl half his age. She loved him and wanted to marry him, but at home his mother objected in her quiet, insistent, passive way. The man felt so guilty that he was finally unable to leave his mother. He didn't return to his lover in Thailand. He died the next year of brain cancer, his doctoral dissertation left unfinished. Why did the cancer strike his brain? Was that the "target organ"—the bodily symbol of his loss?

I remembered Dr. McCullough telling me about a friend of his, a colleague at Yale-New Haven Hospital, an expert in liver surgery who died of liver cancer. Why?

I'd met a woman, a former breast cancer patient who was my mentor and friend while I trained to become a volunteer for the Reach to Recovery Program. She'd had her mastectomy ten years earlier, and when I met her, had recovered from cancer. She was a vivacious enthusiastic woman, married to a reserved man who was more retiring than his outgoing wife, removed, it seemed to me, from her and her great energy.

My friend had two daughters. The older one was a shy, homely, sweet woman with three children. The other daughter was beautiful, talented and vivacious, and she was fifteen years younger than her sister. She was a university student in her senior year, majoring in drama. She dreamed of going to New York and becoming an actress when she graduated.

My friend came down with cancer again, this time of the uterus. Her older daughter nursed her through her long illness. The younger daughter had graduated from college and was now in New York, just starting a promising career as an actress, singer and dancer. After a brave struggle, my friend, their mother, died, and their father remarried. My friend had been dead for a year when the older daughter's husband deserted her, leaving her with the three young children to raise by herself. Soon after, she was diagnosed with breast cancer.

The younger daughter put her career in New York on hold and returned home to care for her sister and the three little ones. The older sister died within months, less than a year after her mother. I went to the funeral. The church was packed with relatives and friends.

The beautiful younger sister, the actress, followed her sister's coffin down the center aisle of the church carrying her little nephew in her arms. She wore a sweater and a long straight skirt with a slit up the side that revealed her shapely dancer's legs. Her two small nieces walked close to her, clutching either side of her skirt as they followed their mother's coffin. The younger sister rose to deliver the eulogy.

"My sister always said that I was the one with the beauty and talent but she was the one with the brains. She told me she was smart enough to know that I was the only one who could raise her children."

At the end of the mass, the children and their beautiful young aunt came sorrowfully up the center aisle and stood at the back of the church as the mourners filed past them. I waited to speak to this girl whose dreams seemed to be lost, the life she wished for over. I was afraid for her. I wanted to tell her what I'd learned, that the depressed spirit can depress one's health, that one must have hope to live. "Remember to take care of yourself! Be strong! Think ahead!" The young woman looked at me as if she couldn't comprehend what I was saying. "Yes," she said. "Of course."

She went back to New York, gathered her belongings and said good-bye to her friends and her career and returned to Florida. She got a job as a high school English teacher and became the second mother to her young nieces and nephew.

My mother's lung cancer began in the same lung that had caused her so much anguish when she was a small child. She'd never smoked a day in her life. She'd always blamed herself for her father's grief at the sight of her, the small, sick child in the hospital. He never came to see her in the hospital again. She went through her life believing she had hurt him terribly. "I made him sad because I was sick!" Was that lung the "target organ" of her cancer, the part of her body that related to the "loss" she'd suffered earlier in her life? Then came the shock of my divorce and the perceived loss of her family and reputation. Could the shame of my divorce have "suffocated" her? Could the loss of her "good name" have taken her breath away? Then came the fatigue, the feeling of helplessness to change the course of events. Six months later, she was dead.

"The cancer patient seems to have been an extrovert, vitally dependent on other persons, other things . . . and when separated from those objects is lost . . . we have found there has been a great mental suffering . . . a total destruction of hope," wrote Elida Evans. "They have started out with full force and it has not been grief alone which stopped them. They have had a peculiar sorrow and a special temperament with which to meet it." Was my mother's "peculiar sorrow" the perceived loss of her reputation?

One of my "sorrows" was that I thought that I'd robbed her of the approval she lived for. My mother and I saw our losses through the prism of our "special temperaments." We were frightened, fragile woman, desperate for approval, who believed we were powerless. Thus began the downward spiral that depressed the immune system and allowed the cancer to grow.

The more I listened to the women I was visiting, the more I read about the disease and the more I thought about my mother's death, the more I understood that I hadn't caused her cancer. My mother could never overcome the lessons she had learned from her father, who had been as fearful and powerless as she. In the end, her fears and beliefs crippled her, betrayed her and led her to her "special temperament" of despair. I was learning so many things that I wished I could tell her. "Be strong within yourself! Don't let anyone have power over you again!"

In his book, *Love, Medicine and Miracles*, Bernie Siegel wrote, "Exceptional patients manifest the will to live in its most potent form. They take charge of their lives even if they were never able to before and they work hard to achieve health and peace of mind . . . If a 'miracle' such as a permanent remission of cancer happens once, it is valid and must not be dismissed as a fluke. If one patient can do it, there's no reason others can't." The book was about his experiences with a therapy group he'd formed called Exceptional Cancer Patients. This was the same group he'd asked me to join. He discovered that exceptional patients see their illness is, as Elida Evans observed, "a warning to take another road." They take responsibility for their own past actions, and most important, they learn how to forgive themselves and others. Through his work with the group, he saw that once exceptional cancer patients learned how to rely on themselves for strength, they refused to be victims, and they realized that they can control their destinies. He was writing about the very lessons he encouraged me to learn in the hospital! The book was a bestseller.

In his second book, *Peace, Love and Healing*, he wrote about people he calls "self induced healers" who have overcome their cancers. "An existential shift has occurred in them, and for the first time in their lives they are truly living," he writes. "They don't see their disease as a sentence but a new beginning . . . I believe that studying the lives of these self-induced healers should be an important part of the attempt first to verify, then to identify the ties between mind and body, psyche and soma. We should know the person as well as the disease and take a special interest in those people who have gotten well despite the odds. They are not just lucky. They have worked hard to achieve their healings and we have much to learn from them."

I read and reread that book many times. I wanted to share what I'd learned from Bernie with the women I was visiting. They were frightened and hurt, and even though many of the women I met seemed to have lost their hope, I wanted them to know me and know that I'd healed myself. So I listened, and I persevered.

CHAPTER TWENTY-THREE

A Vast, Empty Space

Late one night in early November 1989, the phone rang in our apartment in Fort Lauderdale. Pat answered. Peggy and Dennis were calling from his ranch in Montana. I got on the other phone.

"Mom!" she said, with great excitement. "Mom! Dennis and I are getting married!"

"Oh!" I said. "I'm so very happy for both of you! When?"

"Next summer! Out here at the ranch."

They invited us to the ranch for that Thanksgiving. In the few weeks before we went, I found every old family photograph I could and had copies made. There were pictures of my grandparents and my great-grandparents, of my mother and father, of Harry and me shortly after we were married. There was a picture of Peggy, at one year old, a beautiful blonde baby girl with a wistful smile, wearing a baby dress of white organdy. There was a picture of Peggy and her brother and sisters sitting together, taken when she was six, Dana seven, Andrew three and Annie one year old. Peggy and Dana were wearing black velvet dresses with lace collars; Andrew wore short pants and a sweater his grandmother knitted for him. Annie wore the same white organdy baby dress that had been Peggy's. I arranged all the pictures in an album and enclosed a card wishing her and Dennis every happiness as they began their own family.

They were going to Europe after Thanksgiving. The Berlin wall was coming down that fall, and the communist world was collapsing. Dennis wanted to visit Berlin and the Brandenburg Gate, and Peggy wanted to revisit Florence. Pat and I had spent the summer of 1984 in that city, and we'd visited many times since. We had good friends there and I thought that Peggy and Dennis might visit them and that their visit to Florence would be easier for that. I arranged an address book for them with our friends' names and phone numbers and called ahead telling them to expect my daughter and her fiancé.

Peggy picked us up in Bozeman on the day before Thanksgiving, and we drove across bare, brown, windswept plains out to Dennis's ranch. This landscape was different from the gentle wooded hills of New England with small, old towns tucked close to one another. It was a vast land that stretched in sweeping vistas to far away snow-capped mountain ranges.

Dennis was building his dream house, a huge log cabin on the banks of a broad creek. The floors hadn't been laid but the subflooring was down and covered with area rugs. Workmen were busy completing the kitchen, struggling to hook up the dishwasher, stove and refrigerator when we arrived. There was no furniture in the house. It was still in a truck parked in the yard, a barren, treeless space littered with scraps of lumber. Across the yard from the house was a smaller cabin where Dennis and Peggy had been staying while the house was being finished. On the far side of the yard was a one-room guest cottage.

Peggy showed us through the spacious new house. I gave her the album I'd brought from home for her and a small gift for her birthday, which had fallen the week before. She was thrilled with the album and the pictures of her great-grandmother and great-grandfather and of the generations down to her own. "Now you can show these to your own children one day," I said.

We were admiring the great stone fireplace when Dennis hurried in with his mother, Nita, a quiet, slender blonde woman. He introduced Nita and me, then he stepped back as if to admire both of us.

"Don't they look cute together?" he said. Then, as if he'd forgotten something, he turned to Pat. "Pat! Can you help me move some furniture in here?" He looked over at Peggy.

"Sorry, Meg!"

Dennis was thinner than I remembered. His face was flushed and he seemed twitchy and agitated. He was sweating. His clothes were filthy, as if he hadn't changed them in days. I wondered if he was ill. I was surprised to learn that Peggy had arranged rooms for Pat and me at a small lodge and resort, Chico Hot Springs, in a little town called Pray some miles back down the road.

"We'll meet you there for dinner," she said and gave us the keys to one of the cars parked in the yard. We loaded in our bags and headed off.

"Who's staying in that guest house?" said Pat.

"Someone named Bob Seger," I said. "A rock singer."

"Why aren't you staying there?" he said. "You're her mother."

"I don't know."

"Why are we staying miles away from here?"

"I don't know."

The car was an expensive, new, black BMW sedan. Cigarette butts and ashes spilled out of the ashtrays. The dashboard, of burled wood, was scarred with cigarette burns. Empty beer cans, wads of used Kleenex and more cigarette butts covered the floor and the back seat. It belched black smoke as we drove.

"This is a beautiful car," Pat said. "What a shame."

Later the next morning, Thanksgiving Day, we drove back out to the ranch. Dennis's brother, the actor Randy Quaid, and his wife and Nita were already at the house. Randy was a tall, reserved man with a quiet, gentle manner. He was helping Dennis hook up a large-screen television. Dennis was talking and laughing loudly. Soon other guests began to arrive. The rock singer, Bob Seger came in from the guesthouse. A young, blond man named Patrick, a close friend of Peggy's who worked as a personal assistant to Jane Fonda, drove in from the airport. We all sat looking at the television at the throngs of people massed near the Berlin Wall.

"My mother used to tell us about communist Russia and fallout shelters and nuclear war alerts when all the kids had to hide under their desks at school," said Patrick. "Those must have been scary days. Now they seem to be over for good." He was an engaging, bright young man in his late twenties, about Peggy's age. Pat and I began to talk with him about the mass demonstrations that were happening in Germany and the unrest in Romania. Our conversation turned to western Europe and then to our favorite cities in Italy. Randy and his mother sat without speaking and watched us as we talked. Randy's wife stared silently at the television. Peggy was working quietly by herself in the kitchen. Pat and I and Patrick were the only people talking. I remembered the guests at Dennis's New Year's Eve party the year before and wondered if everyone in the movie business was silent. Except for Patrick, these guests had nothing to say. Did they think they had nothing to offer? Did they have anything to offer? Had they decided to offer nothing? It was exhausting to ponder. Dennis and Bob Seger left the room. I saw them through the window heading for the guesthouse.

"I guess your favorite city is Florence," said Patrick. "You know that city so well. I love it too. Imagine visiting the center of the Renaissance!"

"It is the most civilized place," said Pat. "Florentines have a way of making everything into an art form—bread, wine, even breakfast."

A few minutes later, Dennis rushed into the room holding a dead fish high over his head.

"Meg! Meg! Look what I caught!"

He was excited, red-faced and grinning. Peggy looked at him, dismayed. She glanced quickly at me.

"That fish ain't dead, Dennis," said Randy. "All you did was torture it. Put the thing out of its misery."

Dennis took the fish over to the sink and whacked it once, violently, on the counter. He shoved it into the sink and looked angrily at his brother.

"Dennis," I said. "Look. I brought you some names of people to see in Florence."

I brought the address book and some pictures of friends over to the kitchen counter and spread them out for him to see.

"I don't have time for this!" he said. He was furious now.

He swept the pictures away from him and several fell off the counter. I stooped down to pick them up. He pushed past me roughly and I lost my balance. I grabbed the corner of the counter quickly to steady myself. I saw Pat rise out of his chair. He'd seen the whole exchange. I caught his eye and shook my head at him—no, no, no I silently urged. He sat back down, seething. Dennis stalked out of the kitchen and back over to the guesthouse.

Dinner was to be at five o'clock. Pat and I decided to drive back to our hotel for a rest.

"What's the matter with him?" I said. "He's so nice one minute and the next he seems so angry and annoyed."

"Dennis is a spoiled Hollywood infant," said Pat. "That's what's the matter with him."

"I can't understand it! He's a person like anyone else!"

"No he isn't, Susan. He's a cosseted brat. He doesn't think he's a person like everyone else. He thinks he's different. Special. The people who hire him are ruining him. Now he's ruining himself."

"Oh, my God," I said. "Peggy loves him! She's going to marry him! What will happen?"

"I don't know," said Pat. "But he better not be rude to you again."

"I don't think he means it!" I said. "It isn't natural."

"I don't give a royal rat's ass," said Pat. "I saw what happened. He almost knocked you down. He'd better watch his step."

We drove back out to the ranch later that afternoon. I wanted to help Peggy. There were at least ten for dinner, and I knew that she'd done everything herself. She'd planned the menu, made many of the dishes ahead, and rushed into Bozeman to buy china, silverware and crystal only a few days before. I wondered if that was why she seemed tired and preoccupied. But now everyone there was completely silent. Even Patrick said nothing. The men watched television. Every so often one of them would glance over at Dennis, who seemed moody and sullen. I stood in the kitchen trying to make conversation with Nita and Randy's wife. Finally I gave up. Thanksgiving dinner was a wordless affair. Only Dennis spoke, and then just for brief spurts. He seemed to exhaust himself after a few sentences. He left the table several times with Bob Seger and went outside. Each time they came back, Dennis was flushed and jittery.

When the dinner was finally over he suggested that some of us drive up to an old cabin that had once belonged to the legendary film director, Sam Peckinpah. Peggy, Dennis, Pat and I climbed into an old Jeep and drove up the side of one of the foothills behind the house. Dennis drove. At the top we stopped and got out to admire the view for several minutes. As we climbed back in for the ride down, Dennis suddenly reached under the seat of the Jeep, pulled out a pistol and fired it twice into the air. Pat and I jumped.

"Hey, Pat! You're not scared, are ya? It's just a little pistol!"

He jammed the Jeep into first gear and sped down the side of the hill. The Jeep kicked up loose stones and dirt and skidded dangerously on the side of the unpaved road. I was frightened.

"Dennis! Dennis! Please slow down!"

I saw him grinning at me in the rearview mirror.

"Mom! You ain't scared now, are ya? Don't you worry! I'm a great driver, right Meg?"

Peggy said nothing. She sat in the passenger seat and stared out the window. We reached the bottom of the hill, and Dennis gunned the Jeep even faster across the unpaved road to the ranch. Pat and I went into the house, said our good-byes and drove back to our hotel room. I sat down on the bed and cried.

"I can't understand it," I said. "Why doesn't anyone speak? What is wrong?"

"I don't know," said Pat.

We decided to spend the next day at the lodge. I called Peggy to tell her, and I wasn't surprised that she sounded relieved. She called later in the day to say that she and Dennis and some local friends would come to the restaurant to meet us for a last dinner before we went back to Fort Lauderdale.

"If Dennis doesn't behave himself, I'll leave the table," I told Pat. " I refuse to sit through another one of his adolescent snits."

"What about Peggy?"

"I'll explain it to her later," I said.

At dinner, Dennis seemed sheepish and subdued. He insisted on making me his version of a martini.

"This is the Quaid martini!" he announced as he set it down in front of me. "Go ahead, Mom. Take a sip!"

"Thank you, Dennis," I said.

I sipped the martini. It had a burning, fishy taste, and it was very strong. I knew I couldn't finish it.

"How is it?"

"It's fine," I lied. "It's unusual, Dennis. What's in it?"

"Well, vodka, a little vermouth, Tabasco sauce and a couple of anchovies!"

I nodded and smiled.

"Thanks," I repeated.

Later in the dinner, the conversation turned again to the events in Europe. Peggy thanked me again for the names of my friends in Florence. She was looking forward to seeing Berlin.

"We'll bring you back a piece of that old Wall!" Dennis said. He noticed that I hadn't touched my drink. "Why look! That's warm now! You need a chilled one!"

"No, thank you, Dennis. I think it's just a bit too strong."

"I'll fix another one!"

"No, really, Dennis!" I said. "Thank you anyway."

But he'd already scrambled out of his chair. He came back minutes later, flushed and grinning. I saw one of Dennis's friends glance up at him, then shake his head. Then the friend looked back down at his plate. Dennis rapped his fork on his glass as if calling for attention.

"The trouble with all these European dictators is that people take them seriously!" he announced.

"Dennis, people usually take dictators seriously," I said. "It's the people's trouble, not the dictators."

Everyone laughed but Dennis. He scowled at me, red-faced. I saw immediately that he was annoyed. I looked at Pat. We both stood up.

"Peg," I said, "we're going to make this an early night. We'll drive out to say good-bye before we leave."

My daughter wasn't looking at me. She was looking up at Pat, mouth open and eyes wide with terror. I had never seen her look so afraid.

"Peg! What's the matter?" I said.

"Nothing, Mom," she whispered. "Nothing. Good night."

The next day we drove out early to say good-bye. Peggy met us outside the house. Dennis was nowhere in sight. The three of us stood in the yard for a moment, and then Pat went to the car and got in. I remember that November morning in 1989. I remember that it was a November morning like the morning my mother died. It was cold and gray, and a light dust of snow covered the bare ground. I kissed my daughter good-bye. I remember that her cheek was very cold. "I love you, Peggy," I said. She looked at me for a long moment. I remember that there was no expression at all on her face, nothing at all behind her eyes. "I know you do, Mom. I love you, too. Good-bye."

As we pulled away I looked back to see her again. She stood by herself in the dirt yard staring after our car. I saw the distant mountain ranges behind her and the bare, brown plains that surrounded her. I saw my daughter standing by herself in that vast, empty space. I leaned out the window and blew another kiss to her. She stood motionless. I haven't seen her since.

CHAPTER TWENTY-FOUR

Losing Peggy

On the way home to Florida, I couldn't stop asking questions. I could not understand any of what had happened.

"Why did Dennis act that way?"

"I told you. He's an infant."

"Why was she so frightened when she looked at you in that restaurant?"

"Because she knows what I see."

"What's that?"

"Two things. Dennis is an asshole, and she's not going to get the approval she wants from you."

I said nothing further to Pat or anyone else, but I was consumed with worry for days afterward. Who would know the answers to my questions? Finally I called a good friend, a physician in Miami.

"I was visiting some people recently," I said. And then I described Dennis's behavior.

"Who is this person?"

"Just someone we met."

"What you're describing can represent a very serious drug addiction."

"Oh my God! To what?"

"Susan, don't you know anything at all about cocaine?"

"No. I wouldn't know cocaine if I tripped over it."

He laughed.

"Unless there was a mountain of it, I don't think you could trip over it."

"Can he overcome this?"

"From what you've described, I'd say he has a strong addiction. He can overcome it, but it will be very difficult."

I hung up the phone and burst into tears. What could I do? I had no idea. I resolved to say nothing to anyone until I could figure out a way to proceed. Just before Christmas an envelope from the Hotel Ritz in Paris arrived. Inside was a check from Peggy for thirty-three hundred dollars made out to me and a small piece of blue painted concrete—a piece of the Berlin Wall. "Peace on earth!" The card read. "Merry, merry Christmas, Love, Meg and Dennis." It was the first time she'd ever signed her name as "Meg." I called several times to talk to her and thank her, but I couldn't reach her. Christmas Day came and went without a call from her. When I finally did hear from her in February, she was as cool and remote as she'd been the last time I'd seen her, and the call was short, obligatory.

"Is everything okay, Peg?" I said.

"Yes, Mom! Why do you ask?" She sounded irritated and impatient.

I couldn't bring myself to say anything about my worry.

One morning, the next month, in March 1990, I picked up the newspaper and read that following the premiere of Peggy's new movie, *Joe Versus the Volcano,* in New York, Dennis threw popcorn all over a hotel lobby and had tried to kick a photographer. Peggy had screamed for him to stop. The news article said that she'd burst into tears. I put the paper down.

"That's it," I said to Pat. "I have to call her."

I picked up the phone and dialed her number. I told her what I'd read.

"I'm very worried about you," I said. "I have been for some time. I feel that I have to ask you this. Does Dennis have a problem with cocaine?"

"It's really not something I want to talk about, Mom." Suddenly she burst into tears. "I have to go," she said and hung up.

She didn't call me for months after that. I tried to reach her, left messages, but she didn't return my calls until a month before the wedding was to take place.

Her wedding was set for July at the ranch in Montana. It was to be a big barbecue to which all the members of both families had been invited. I'd been getting phone calls from people representing "Parties Plus," who said they were doing "the Meg-Dennis wedding." They begged me not to reveal the date and location of the wedding.

"Who would I say anything to?" I asked one of them.

"Paparazzi! The press! Meg and Dennis don't want their wedding ruined."

"I don't know any paparazzi. It's a private affair. Why would I tell anyone?"

"Everything is going to be booked under the name Marvin Hooperman. But don't breathe a word!"

Several weeks before the wedding, most of the people in our family had been invited. My father, my brothers, my sister and her family were all flying out from Connecticut. Andrew and Annie had formed a band and were singing together in Atlanta where they now lived. They were flying out to the ranch. The only people who, inexplicably hadn't been invited were Dana and her husband, now stationed in California.

Dana called me one morning, wondering.

"Did I say anything to upset her, Mom?"

"I'm sure it was an oversight," I told her. "Maybe she doesn't have your address."

I called Peggy.

"Oh, gee," she said. "I'll have someone call her right away. Do you have her number?"

"Peg, can't you call your sister? I think she'd like to talk to you. She's worried she offended you in some way and that's why she didn't get an invitation."

"Mom, I don't think you understand how big my life is right now," she said crisply. "I'll have someone call her."

"I keep talking to these assistants. Don't you want to talk to me about your wedding?"

"Mom," she said patiently. "You and I don't have that kind of relationship." I was stunned. Confused again. Had I missed something? What? When?

"What do you mean?" I said. She didn't answer.

"I have to go, Mom. Really, I have so much to do." Then she hung up. Later that afternoon she called me back.

"Mom, please don't criticize me about the people who are helping me with my wedding. I need their help. You couldn't possibly know what kind of a life I have."

"I didn't criticize you," I said. "I wondered why I talk to your assistants and not you about your wedding. And I asked you to call your sister."

"Mom, I can't be bothered with all this right now! It's so petty."

"It's not petty when someone's feelings are hurt, even by accident."

"Do you know how petulant you're being?" She paused. "And what is this that you think Dennis is a drug addict?" This last question she screamed out at me furiously.

"Peg! I never said he was a drug addict! I asked you if he had a problem with cocaine!"

"What do you even know about drugs?"

"I don't know anything. That's why I was asking."

"Who are you to ask me these things?" She was screaming into the phone.

"I'm your mother." It was the only thing I could think of to say.

"How dare you say anything like this to me!"

"Because I love you," I said. Now I was angry. "And I might be one of the few people who dares to tell you the truth!"

She slammed down the phone. Later that night she called me back.

"Mom, the wedding's off."

"Oh my goodness," I said. "Peg, wait a minute." But it was too late. She'd hung up. She has not spoken to me since.

Several days after that phone call, in late June 1990, Dennis checked himself into a drug rehabilitation program at St. John's hospital in Santa Monica, California. My sister called to tell me that Peggy was telling the press she had no idea that Dennis had a drug addiction.

"How could she live with him all those months and not know that?" my sister asked.

"I don't know."

"Did you know?"

"No. I just thought something was wrong. I didn't know what it was."

ᕈᕈᕈᕈᕈ

There was much I didn't know. In the weeks and months that followed, I heard nothing about Peggy. And then a strange silence descended over my entire family. My other children wouldn't tell me anything about her. I asked Annie.

"Meg doesn't want you to know anything about her, Mom. She doesn't want to hear anything about you."

I asked Andrew.

"I can't involve myself in this, Mom."

"But you have her number! You see her!"

"She doesn't want to hear about you. I can't intrude on that."

One day, in spring 1991, waiting in line at the grocery store, I read in *People* magazine that Peggy and Dennis had married on Valentine's Day in California. Why had no one told me?

And then I began to read about myself in magazines and newspapers. One Sunday morning, I picked up the newspaper and read, "Meg Ryan refuses to speak to the mother who abandoned her." I was shocked. I had never abandoned my children! Soon other stories about me and my daughter began to pour forth. In the following weeks and months, magazines like *Redbook, Good Housekeeping, Vanity Fair* and *People* retold the same story. There were elaborations: Meg Ryan's mother had "abandoned" her children, "walked out of her marriage to pursue an acting career in New York City." I was no longer the "much-admired mother." I was the shallow woman who "walked out on her family to pursue ill-advised dreams of fame and stardom." I was no longer Peggy's "schoolteacher mother." I'd become a "failed actress." Peggy's "happy" childhood was now "thirty-two years of stuff with this woman." "Susan drove off in her old Ford Pinto, bound for Manhattan, and a career, she hoped, in regional theatre. Harry was left to tend to the four children." "Meg Ryan describes the pain of her mother's abandonment as 'a motivator for my career.'" How could magazines print such irresponsible things? Who could have told them such blatant lies?

A few days later, a friend called to tell me that a cover story about Peggy had appeared in *People* magazine and that I should read it. I went down to the drugstore and bought the magazine. "A happy marriage and a new baby help heal the wounds of a long rift with her mother," blared the headline. I hadn't even known she was pregnant.

Then I read that Peggy had instructed her family not to give me her phone number or address. I called Harry.

"Did you tell them I abandoned them? That I drove away because I wanted to be an actress?"

"Of course not."

"Is this true that she told everyone not to give me her phone number or address?"

"Yes. She forbade it. She was adamant."

"What do you mean 'forbid'? She can't control you! You're her father!"

"She said if I gave it to you she would change her number and not give it to me. She said not to speak to the press."

"Harry! If no one else in our family speaks out then the lies go on!" I was heartsick. What had happened to my daughter? How could she behave this way? Each time one of Peggy's movies came out the story reappeared. Try as I would to overcome my shock and embarrassment, I couldn't. I began to get phone calls from old friends in Connecticut.

"Susan, how can Peggy lie about you?"

"I don't know." I was devastated.

I asked Pat. "Why does she lie about me?"

"It's called spin, Susan. Damage control. You're the first casualty. Don't you see that she's protecting her image?"

"But why would she use me to do that?"

"She thought you'd tell the world about Dennis's drug problem."

"But I didn't do that!"

"She thought you would. So to cut you off, she discredits you. She tells the media you were the shallow, failed actress mother who walked out on her kids for a career that didn't work out. Now the public won't believe a thing you say about Dennis or anything else."

"Why would she do such a thing?"

"She's trying to control you. You don't see that."

"Why does she say I was a failed actress when she never even mentioned I was an actress before! I used to think that was so strange! Why does she say it now in such a negative way?"

"To diminish you. To trivialize you."

"But why?"

"She's not like most daughters. She doesn't want to be like her mother. She wants to be her mother. She wants her mother to be someone else. Someone less."

"How could anyone not want me to be me?" I simply couldn't understand it.

The silence in my family grew ever deeper. I read about her little boy, my grandson, in magazines. Unexpectedly, former nannies who'd read that I'd never seen my grandson sent me pictures of him as a toddler at two and three. They extended sympathy and insisted on anonymity. Only Dana sent me a picture of him . . . as a little boy of four. He looked like his mother when she was his age. He had the same blond hair, the same pale, blue eyes, the same winsome smile. I began looking for other pictures of him in the magazines.

As the years passed and Peggy became more famous, the stories about our estrangement seemed to take on a distorted energy of their own. I began to dread the release of any of her movies. I knew there would be yet another interview about the devastation I had caused her.

No one in my family would come forward to defend me. I asked them why. The answers were the same. "I don't want to get involved. I don't want to be a public person." I didn't want to be a public person either. But suddenly I was. And I was angry. Against my will, I found myself in the glare of a public spotlight, falsely portrayed as a mother who had abandoned her children to pursue a career as an actress. My daughter's public relations representatives promulgated the lie about me. It flooded through magazine racks and over television gossip shows and soon became embedded in the public record. My daughter never disavowed the lie. Instead, she refused to speak about me, forbade others in my family to speak about me and I was left, slandered, with no way to defend myself. I had no public relations firm to tell the truth for me. When, finally, reporters did call me and I tried to defend myself, they never printed my protestations; they never printed what I told them had really happened. They needed Meg Ryan's image for future covers. They didn't need her mother's truths.

Slowly, I began to realize that my daughter was forcing me to confront my weakness, the old childhood lesson I thought I'd overcome—fear of disapproval. I still had to fight that fear. But I did not feel guilty. I knew who I was. In the end, I understood that my daughter's actions were her own. I might never understand them. But I would not succumb to shame for something I didn't do even though the world might think I had. What was I going to do . . . follow my mother and my grandfather into the grave because of a lost reputation? Hadn't I learned anything? I would not lose my balance . . . capsize . . . go down. I forgave my daughter and I went on.

One year Pat was given a magazine assignment to profile Bobby Drinnon, a well-known psychic, a man famous for his work helping police solve criminal cases and also famous for advising celebrities and movie stars. Pat was leaving for rural Tennessee to interview him. At the last minute, I went with him. We met Bobby and his wife for dinner at a local restaurant in the town near his home. He was a small, gentle man with shoulder-length white hair, ethereally white skin and the round pudgy face of an aged angel. He had no idea who I was, only that I was the wife of the writer who had come there to interview him. We sipped glasses of wine and ordered our dinners and Pat began his interview. Suddenly the little man stopped speaking in mid-sentence, reached across the table and took my hand. "I'm so very sorry," he said. "You have lost a child."

I was shocked. I knew all my children were safe.

"No," I said. "My children are safe."

"Oh?" he said in his gentle voice. "But one is missing."

I looked at Pat who was as confused as I. I said nothing.

The next day I went with Pat to the man's house. Just before we left I told him that he was right. I had lost my daughter. Briefly, I told him the story. "How did you know?" I asked him.

"I can see auras around people," he said. "Hazy, colored circles of energy that surround people and reflect who they are . . . their life-spirit, if you like. Yours is blue, a violet blue. And a big piece of it is missing."

⊙⊙⊙⊙⊙

A few years later, I was waiting at an intersection in Fort Lauderdale for a red light to change to green. A bus rolled by in front of me with my daughter's picture pasted on the side of it. As I sat staring, her face glided past me, larger than life. Her name was under the picture. Meg Ryan. A movie star! It dawned on me, at that moment, why for all these years people have asked me what it's like to be the mother of a movie star. I am the mother of a movie star. But I only read about the mothers of other movie stars. I don't know what they know. I know what it is like to go to the grocery store and pick up a newspaper and read how my daughter, the movie star, said that I abandoned her to become a failed actress. I know what it's like to see my daughter's picture in *Vanity Fair* magazine and read that what I thought was a loving relationship between us has become "thirty-two years of stuff with this woman." I know what it's like to look at her face on one of those covers and try to find somewhere, in the picture of this woman who is now Meg, the baby, the little girl, the young woman, my child, my daughter, Peggy, who I loved. I don't know who she has become.

I know that my daughter has excluded me from her life and that even as I write this, I don't know why. I can only guess. Maybe she was afraid I would discover Dennis's drug problem? That I might discover something about her she didn't want me to know? That there was something about me . . . my "self" that disturbed her? Was Pat right, after all, when he said, "She doesn't want to be like you, she wants to be you, and she wants you to be someone else . . . someone less." But I can't do that. Not even for her.

EPILOGUE

Pat and I bought our own house here in Fort Lauderdale several years ago. It's an old wooden house near the beach. It was built in 1928 right after a big hurricane blew through here, and it's been through some big storms since. It has overhanging eaves and gables and a long row of windows in back that face east, toward the ocean. It looks like a little New England beach house except that we painted it pink and white. It has a tin roof, a picket fence, palm trees and a rose hibiscus out front.

We used to ride by this house on our bicycles. Something about it always seemed to call out to us. We rode by for months before we summoned our courage, knocked on the front door and asked the lady who owned it if she'd sell it to us. She did.

We spent months taking moldering plaster off the walls and ceilings and exposed the old Dade County red pine beams. We took down partition walls that tenants had put up over the years and gave the house back the airy space it had when it was first built. We pulled up old linoleum and found red pine floors. We pulled cracked tile down in the bathroom and discovered a big, old oval tub with claw feet. We painted the floor under it a pale, sea green and we imagine that we're bathing in the ocean. We pried open all the paned windows so the sunlight floods in and the sea breezes blow through our little wooden house, giving it new life.

We're filling the house with Haitian art, vibrant images of emerald-green fish and teal-blue mermaids and happy people in outdoor markets. The people are buying red and yellow mangoes and papaya and deep violet flowers. A black tin figure of a Haitian girl stands on a shelf in the front hall facing the front door. Her arms are outstretched in greeting.

We have six dogs now. Stella had two puppies that we wouldn't give up. Our dogs lay sprawled around the house like red and black rugs, worn out from playing in the sun, chasing lizards. One of the young ones, Sweetness, will try to grab a nap on the new sofa in the sunroom. He sleeps with his head under a pillow. He thinks if he doesn't see us then we aren't there to shoo him off.

The late-afternoon sun plays on the white birdcage that belongs to our little, yellow parakeet, Francis. I named him for Saint Francis of Assisi, the patron saint of birds and animals. I learned his prayer years ago, and some of the lines have special resonance for me today. "For it is by giving that we receive; it is by losing that we find; it is by forgiving that we are forgiven." That is what the animals in their simplicity do. They teach us always about the power of love and forgiveness. My dogs know how to give without giving themselves away. They forgive without reservation or judgment. And I know that it is by losing that we find. I know that thoughts can heal and that there is no more powerful thought than the healing thought of forgiveness.

My bird sits on top of his cage; he doesn't like being in it. He looks golden in the sunlight. I hold my finger out to him, and he hops on it, then he cocks his head sideways, staring at me intently with his beady, little black eyes. He starts to cluck and scold and then he lets out that long whistle he makes before he says something to me.

"Kiss me!" he shrieks. "I love you! I'm a beautiful bird!"

My grandmother's clock stands in the corner of our living room. Its soft, silver chimes still sound every precious quarter-hour. They remind me of that long-ago night when the same chimes woke me in her house. I remember her pale, blue eyes and her hand holding mine. I remember her words: "Remember, dear girl. You always have yourself." In those days, I didn't know what she meant. Now I know that if you live for others' approval you give up yourself.

Outside my window the leaves of the huge, old gumbo limbo tree that shades our house flutter in the sea wind, and I can hear the faint sound of wind chimes and tamarinds that we hung high on one of its branches. In the late afternoon, flocks of bright green parrots squawk and cackle at one another in those branches. Above the tree, high in the clear sky, I can see the sunlight flash on a silver plane coming in to Fort Lauderdale. Pat's oldest son is on the plane with his wife and little boy, Pat's grandson. He's a sturdy two-year-old with red hair, curious and determined. He'll do what he usually does when he stays at our house. He'll go to the drawer under the stove and take out every pot and pan. He'll bring them to every corner of the house and put them in piles and bang them together. The dogs will eye him wearily and find their own corners, away from the noise. Pat will call out from his office, the clacking of his typewriter muted by the clanging of the pots and pans. "Hey! Testa Rosa! Redhead! Stop banging the pots!" I pick him up and carry him to the piano and place his chubby little fingers on the keys.

"See?" I say to him. "This is a beautiful noise. This is a noise you can control!" He looks up at me, surprised and delighted, and we pick out the notes of one of his nursery songs. "Ah," says Pat. "That's better." Even the dogs look satisfied.

I think back to when I was a little girl, a child of five, terrified of noises in the night, the sound of a plane roaring over my head in the darkness, terrified of the unexpected and desperately trying to find a place to hide. There is no need to hide from fear and fright now. I've learned that I'm not helpless, that I can face my fears and overcome them. I think about the cancer I once had, and I know that if, as some have said, cancer represents loss, then recovery is gain. I've

gained so much since those days when I was a small girl beating on the door of our apartment in the night, trying to find a safe place to hide from what might happen. Now I know that the safest, brightest place is within myself.

Now I know that the lessons we learn and the patterns we form in childhood can overcome the spirit and lead to that "special temperament" of despair. It is the small betrayal of self over the years, the giving up of little bits and pieces of the self, the loss of self-strength that leads to fear. Then comes the downward spiral toward hopelessness, despair and death.

I remember my mother. I planted a gardenia bush in the front yard in her memory. Gardenias were her favorite flowers. She is buried on the side of a gentle hill in a cemetery in New York state. Standing next to her gravestone, you can see the broad sweep of a valley and in the far distance, the purple rolling hills of Connecticut resting in the sun. On her gravestone is written: "Beloved, if God has so loved us, we also ought to love one another." In the end, she left a far sweeter lesson than her fear.

And, as always, I remember my grandmother. I can still see her, striding down the avenue at seventy, head high, determined not to miss the train to the ballgame. I can just hear her, calling back over her shoulder to her family, "What are you worried about? Of course I'm going! I'm in charge. I can take care of myself!"

On my desk I have framed some lines from a poem by Samuel Hazo called, "The First and Only Sailing."

To live
You leave your yesterselves
To drown without a funeral.
You chart a trek where no
One's sailed before.
You rig. You anchor up. You sail.

Sometimes I see myself as I was at twelve, a skinny girl, dark hair tied in pigtails, straining at the rudder and pulling at the sail of that old, wooden boat. I am, as she was, still tacking into the wind, still trying not to be blown over by guilt or shame. I try not to be overcome by my weaknesses and fears. I don't want to capsize and go down. I struggle always to keep my balance. For me, to live is like sailing in rough weather. It's in my nature to be fearful. But I know that if I am prepared, if I know this truth about myself, I can take the rudder with a firm hand, ride over the wave of fear, come out on the other side and be ready for the next one. I chose a new course. I am the sailor. It's my boat. For those who will choose a new way, know that sometimes no one wants to travel with you. You forgive them and forgive yourself and go on alone. I remember the poet Seneca. He wrote: "Fear leads toward death. Courage leads to the stars." I have learned the truth of that.